PROBLEM MANAGEMENT IN
ENDOCRINE SURGERY

PROBLEM MANAGEMENT IN ENDOCRINE SURGERY

GLENN W. GEELHOED, M.D.

Associate Professor of Surgery
Chief, Transplantation Division
Director, Surgical Research Laboratories
and Surgical Endocrinology Service
George Washington University Medical Center
Washington, D.C.

YEAR BOOK MEDICAL PUBLISHERS, INC.

CHICAGO • LONDON

Library of Congress Cataloging in Publication Data

Geelhoed, Glenn W.
Problem management in endocrine surgery.

Includes index.
1. Endocrine glands—Surgery. 2. Endocrine glands—Diseases. I. Title. [DNLM: 1. Endocrine glands—Surgery. WK 100 G297p]
RD599.G43 1982 617'.44 82-10850
ISBN 0-8151-3412-6

For
DONALD WILLIAM
and
MICHAEL ALAN

Contents

Foreword

In this volume Dr. Geelhoed has concentrated on one aspect of the surgical management of a whole series of diseases and disorders. This is not a book on "diagnosis" or "pre- and postoperative care" or "operative technique." Instead, it concentrates on the events immediately surrounding the operation and, in certain instances, some of the newer aspects of diagnosis that might be carried out by quasioperative means (e.g., transhepatic sampling of the portal vein). Several of the procedures should properly be carried out either in the operating room or close to the time and place of operation: they are "perioperative" diagnostic methods.

As in any book dealing with operations performed by highly specialized surgeons, the object is not to guide the inexperienced by cookbook procedures, taking the surgeon by the hand through procedures he may never see or do again. If a book on surgical management in specialized areas ever has such an object, it is being published 30 years too late.

Instead, this book recognizes that in every major center of the country there will be 3 or 4 people who concentrate on some of the rare endocrine neoplasms and possibly 40 or 50 who deal with the other, commoner disorders. It is to those surgeons, and to those students of surgery, interns, or residents who are pointing in that direction, that this book speaks.

Its usefulness will be found not only in guidance to better and safer surgical care, but also in the stimulus it may give to others to provide alternative opinions, or record in the literature the outcome of experiences conducted by alternative means.

Dr. Geelhoed is to be congratulated on completing this remarkable volume. May it have a long and useful life, passing through future editions as this rapidly changing field further evolves.

Francis D. Moore, M.D.
Elliott Carr Cutler Professor of Surgery
Harvard Medical School
Boston, Massachusetts

Preface

SURGICAL ENDOCRINOLOGY is a dynamic, expanding new discipline. Understanding of neuroendocrine control systems has developed rapidly with the integration of genetic, embryologic, and biochemical information into meaningful patterns. Refined techniques of radioimmunoassay and radiographic imaging have made diagnosis and localization of endocrine hyperfunction much more precise. As a result, surgical treatment can now be guided toward restoring patients to the normal balance of physiologic autoregulation as well as curing them of endocrinologic excess.

Endocrine surgical patients usually seek help for the resolution of problems that are functional; rarely is the mere presence of an endocrine tumor the patient's complaint. In only one anatomical area discussed in this book—the thyroid—is the tumor mass likely to be a problem noted by the patient. More often, *finding* a hidden tumor will be a problem for the physician. However, increasing application of sophisticated imaging techniques on asymptomatic patients has increased the incidental discovery of nonfunctioning masses in endocrine organs. With the exception of these "incidentalomas" that are localized before diagnosis, the increasing sensitivity and specificity of endocrinologic testing can confirm the diagnosis of preclinical disease. When cautiously applied—particularly in stimulation tests for screening family members with hereditable endocrinopathy—endocrine surgery can *prevent* some diseases before they cause patient problems.

This book is designed to deal with endocrine surgical problems: those presented by the patient in the clinical syndromes of their disease, and those posed to the physician in management of the diagnostic and therapeutic options among a sometimes bewildering array of new methods. It is hoped that the text will be useful to the student who is taught by patients, whether he be at an undergraduate, postgraduate, or continuing education level in surgery, medicine, or radiology.

Each chapter begins with the patient's problems as a starting point for the management process by the physician. The tumors, hormones, and syndromes are reviewed as background for a diagnostic approach in screening, confirmation, and localization. Discussion of treatment includes preoperative preparation, anesthesia and operative technique, postoperative care, and follow-up for special consideration of each of the endocrine surgical problems.

Any book dealing with the challenging problems and myriad unanswered questions in a rapidly advancing field will be biased by the prejudices and limited by the experiences of the author at the time it is written. However, the conceptual framework of neuroendocrinology as an integrated physiologic control system can be helpful to the reader in assimilating new information in endocrinology as it develops. It is easier to assay than to understand the abundance of hormones and candidate hormones that are now emerging; but the clinical significance of a patient problem without a known mediator remains more compelling than that of a candidate hormone without a known effect. By observing and listening to our patients' problems we will learn to further modify our concepts and to initiate new procedures in the management of neuroendocrine disorders.

GLENN W. GEELHOED

1 / Introduction: Neuroendocrinology and Endocrine Surgery

Endocrine surgery is physiologic surgery. The endocrine surgeon must recognize the often subtle deviations from normal physiology in the effects of abnormal metabolism in the target end-organ. The metabolic derangements that are the primary problem in surgical endocrinology make this discipline distinctive from most other fields of surgical specialty interest, which often begin with anatomical derangement and "mass lesion" effects. The anatomical abnormality is often inapparent as the endocrine surgeon follows the physiologic clues through the identification of a humoral mediator. The rational inference of an abnormality in this humoral mediator based on the observed clinical findings may lead further to a search for the source of hormonal hyper- or hyposecretion. Observing the effects of the mediator in the clinical syndrome evident through the target organ's reaction leads the physician back primarily to the source of the endocrine secretion. Only then, with diligence in the use of radiologic and operative techniques for localization, does the surgeon encounter the anatomical defect that gave rise to the hormonal imbalance and the clinical syndrome. This discovery of a morphological abnormality in the endocrine surgical patient often requires the pathologist's techniques to confirm subtle variants from normal structure. Endocrine surgery, then, is not so much the surgery of mass lesions and the correction of anatomical defects as the restoration of normal endocrine physiologic balance in functions. Looking forward along the same inferential pathway, this book will discuss each of several endocrine surgical abnormalities from the starting point of the tumor, its hormones, and the clinical syndrome that results.

The myriad and often confusing presentations of patients with hormonal disorders would require a large capacity for rote memory from the clinical observation of these syndromes. A long experience would be required before the difficult integration of much of this clinical information into meaningful patterns might be possible. Fortunately, the details of clinical observation cluster—not randomly, but within recognizable patterns—in the clinical syndromes. Study of hormone origin and function makes the organization of the details of clinical experience much more rational and easier not only in remembering the clinical patterns but also in assimilating new information in endocrinology. The precision of many endocrinologic diagnostic tests, enhanced by radioimmunoassay techniques, has sharpened the clinician's focus on clinical syndromes. New radiologic techniques contribute to a very refined capability to localize subtle morphological abnormalities preoperatively. The organization of diagnostic methods used in this book will proceed from screening methods through confirmation of the endocrine diagnosis to localization techniques (Table 1–1). It is the surgeon's responsibility, then, to correct the disorders of surgical endocrinology by intervening directly and by reducing or ablating endocrine tissue, correcting hyperfunction, removing neoplasm, and restoring the patient, ideally, toward the balance of physiologic autoregulation.

This pattern of behavior in endocrine surgery is generally applicable, but becomes critical in some specific endocrine surgical abnormalities that may be life-threatening. Recognition of these high-risk endocrine abnormalities requires that the surgeon be a capable endocrinologist who can manage the patient problems that result from such life-threatening syndromes. Safety in patient management and judgment in intervention are critically important in endocrine surgery. Preoperative preparation of the patient and details of postoperative management parallel the technical aspects of opera-

TABLE 1–1.—OUTLINE FOR DISCUSSION OF EACH CLINICAL SYNDROME IN THIS BOOK

Management problems
For the patient
For the physician
Introduction to the endocrinologic abnormality
The tumor
The hormone
The syndrome
Diagnosis
Screening
Confirmation
Localization
Preoperative preparation
Anesthesia management
Operative technique
Postoperative care and drug management
Follow-up and special considerations

tive dissection in importance. Kocher's technique of thyroidectomy awaited Plummer's use of iodine before the operation could be safely performed to the benefit of patients with hyperthyroidism. Repletion of contracted blood volume and restoration of electrolyte deficits are major features of the endocrine surgery of several syndromes, rivaling the significance of operative technique. The careful use of blocking agents and proper anesthetic technique are critically important in the management of the patient with pheochromocytoma. A major focus of this book will be on the management of these perioperative problems, including preoperative preparation and anesthesia management (Table 1–1), as well as on operative technique.

Endocrine tumors rarely present solely as mass lesions producing signs and symptoms by impinging upon or growing into adjacent viscera. Endocrine tumors rarely disrupt function by their presence alone. In two instances in this book we will discuss primary lesions simply because they occupy space; one such tumor is in the neck and the other is hidden in the silent suprarenal retroperitoneum. A more common problem in endocrine surgery is locating the source of hormonal hypersecretion. The reverse of symptoms caused by a tumor merely by its mass is the problem in localizing a source of known hypersecretion that may remain obscure even on the operating table with the gland exposed for inspection, palpation, and biopsy examination.

BIOLOGIC CONTROL SYSTEMS AND THEIR IMBALANCE

Biologic control systems are servomechanisms that delicately seek a balance in homeostasis. In the most simple example, a gland secretion, a hormone, exerts an effect upon a target organ, which in turn results in diminished hormonal secretion. The source of such a hormone may not be a single or paired gland: the chromaffin system consists of many nests of cells located throughout the body, and this more diffuse system has broken down the concept of "a ductless gland" as a focal distinctive organ. It is now recognized that a "gland" may not be a group of cells located in a single anatomical site; similar cells may act from widely scattered anatomical locations. For example, different species of pancreatic islets are scattered within an exocrine gastrointestinal (GI) tract gland, and similarly functioning cells may be found outside the pancreas itself.

The body's biologic control systems can be approached either through endocrinology or through the study of a different discipline—neurology. It could be postulated that the CNS is primarily in control of all the activity of the organism's component parts. The CNS transfers information by electric impulse and by neurotransmitters. The belief that the CNS and the endocrine system were independent in exerting control has been confounded by the later discovery that some of these CNS neurotransmitters circulate systemically with hormonal effects, and hormones controlling GI secretion have been found in the CNS acting as neurotransmitters!

Integration of the CNS and peripheral hormonal secretion is accomplished by the ductless messenger system of the hypophysis–pituitary portal venous system. Releasing factors elaborated by the hypophysis transfer information from the CNS to the pituitary gland. The pituitary releases a hormone (ACTH, TSH, and so on) which influences another endocrine gland in the periphery. The peripherally secreted hormone is perceived by the CNS and hypophyseal secretion is shut down, completing the servomechanism loop (Fig 1–1). Further examples of interesting collaboration between these biologic control systems have become more apparent whenever one chooses to study a patient problem as one of purely endocrine or neurologic abnormality.

When interruption of the loop in this neurohumoral servosystem occurs, clinical syndromes of hormonal excess or deficiency result. The precise site of interruption may not be apparent. Cushing's *disease* is based upon excess ACTH production by the CNS; Cushing's *syndrome* results from ex-

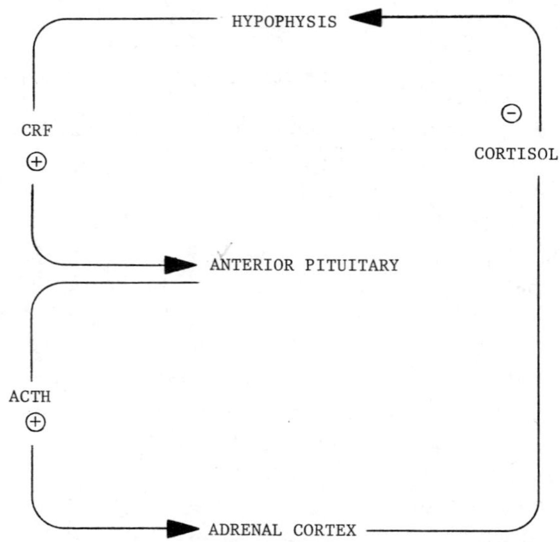

Fig 1–1.—The hypophysis-pituitary-adrenal axis offers a near-perfect example of the integration of neuroendocrine control systems, with neurotransmitters and classic hormones in feedback control of a vital homeostatic system. CRF, corticotropin-releasing factor.

cess cortisol produced by an autonomous adrenal gland. Whether Cushing's syndrome was a neural or humoral loss of control was a question that concerned Harvey Cushing for most of his professional life and remains important today for the differentiation of hypercortisolism. Two patients who exhibit very much the same syndrome can be found to have the origin of this syndrome in quite distant sources: one could say that Cushing's disease is based in a neurologic illness and Cushing's syndrome is based in an autonomous endocrine glandular hyperfunction. However, the effect on patient problems is the same from either source or from exogenous steroid therapy.

The syndromes of hormonal excess are independent of the site of hormone secretion. Patients may exhibit problems based in tumors at different anatomical sites; for example, catecholamine excess produces the same clinical syndrome whether the source of hypersecretion is an adrenal pheochromocytoma or a cervical glomus jugulare tumor. Secretory diarrhea may be a patient's chief complaint, even if the physician discovers that the primary problem is medullary thyroid carcinoma, a carcinoid tumor of the ileum, or a pancreatic islet cell tumor.

Clinical syndromes, therefore, do not always predict the focal pathophysiologic source of disease in endocrine surgery as they often do in other fields of medicine. This factor becomes even more fascinating when it is found that the syndromes may in some instances "cluster" either simultaneously or sequentially within a given patient—and the same or similar syndromes may occur throughout the family of such a patient!

THE APUD CONCEPT

Much of our knowledge of endocrinology has been clarified by the APUD concept. Some of the remarkable coincidences in clinical syndromes may be linked to fundamental processes going on in the cell. The APUD concept is based upon studies of embryology, biochemistry, genetics, and pathophysiology, and explains similarities of endocrine illness resulting from benign and malignant neoplasms occurring at different anatomical sites, as well as multiple endocrine adenopathy (MEA) within a patient and within families.

The unifying concept developed by Pearse[1] evokes "neural crest cell dysplasia" to explain some of the coincidences seen in clinical neuroendocrinology. The neural crest cell is an ectoderm-derived cell which migrates embryonically throughout the body, carrying with it common enzymes, staining characteristics, and endocrine properties. Neural crest cells lose their embryonic association with the CNS and differentiate into the chromaffin system, producing amine hormones, and into the autonomic nervous system. The same cell line may associate with gut endodermal cells in an enterochromaffin system, producing polypeptide hormones.

A common biochemical feature of APUD cells is their capacity for "amine precursor uptake and decarboxylation"; hence the acronym APUD. Descendants of this cell line may synthesize amine hormones or link these amines into polypeptides with hormonal or marker functions. They are highly integrated with the CNS and may exert extracellular feedback upon one another, similar to intracellular enzymatic processes. A single cell line defect may have protean clinical consequences and explain clustering of endocrine abnormalities in a given patient as well as within a family. As our information base expands within endocrinology or within studies of neurotransmitters in the nervous system, many common origins and functions are found within the genetics, embryology, and biochemistry of each system. As this integration of the neurohumoral control systems becomes more apparent, we can say that neuroendocrinology has lost its hyphen.

THE PRECISION OF SURGICAL ENDOCRINOLOGY AND ITS MARKERS

Simultaneously with the evolution of the APUD concept, the techniques of radioimmunoassay emerged. These precise assay techniques allowed the determination of minute hormonal concentrations in cells and in plasma. Suppression and stimulation studies could now be used to measure hormone response directly. Observation of clinical features is a necessary but crude step toward the definition of an endocrine syndrome. With more hormones that can be precisely quantitated in extremely small concentrations, screening and diagnosis have been refined. For many endocrine syndromes, the diagnosis is obtained more safely by suppression than by provocative testing, particularly if hormonal excess can lead to a life-threatening crisis. Very precise low-level radioimmunoassay sensitivity has made suppression testing more useful. The availability of these assays has also defined relationships of complex hormonal disorders, such as those now known to be present in multiple endocrine adenopathy.

With the availability of sophisticated testing and integrating concepts for the pathophysiology of associated endocrine abnormalities, how can we apply these basic advances in management of patient problems? A purpose of this text will be the integration of basic endocrine theory with quantitative biochemical assays in the application of this knowledge to the endocrine surgical patient.

THE PERIOPERATIVE MANAGEMENT OF THE ENDOCRINE SURGICAL PATIENT

Table 1–1 is the outline we will follow in discussing several endocrine surgical syndromes.

The initial points of reference are the patient and his problems, both the symptoms and the signs as experienced by the patient and as witnessed by the physician. The endocrinologic abnormality, including the tumor, the hormones, and the syndromes, are then discussed, and the uses of the laboratory to define the hormonal defects are outlined. After confirmation of the endocrine diagnosis, techniques of anatomical localization are discussed. Preoperative preparation will concentrate on efforts to control the patient's endocrine abnormalities prior to surgical correction. We will discuss selective aspects of intraoperative management, focusing on patient safety in anesthesia management and operative technique. Postoperative care must consider hormonal deficits or residual hyperfunction. Continued observation of the patient is crucial. Also, screening the family of the patient who has a hereditary disorder is the physician's responsibility in follow-up. The dynamism of surgical endocrinology makes completing a book at any one point in time hazardous. I urge the reader to leave open-ended the further evolution of management techniques for problems experienced by these patients in a dynamically developing field in which new concepts are developing almost daily. At the present imperfect state of the art I have personal prejudices and preferences in management that I frankly admit at the outset. The APUD concept itself does not perfectly fit all of the reference standards in endocrine surgery. Patients will continue to educate us through presentation of persistent problems, which will cause further modifications of theory and adaptation of practice. Both conceptual and management frameworks will be undergoing further refinements with the rapid developments and dynamic growth of surgical endocrinology.

REFERENCE

1. Pearse A.G.E.: The cytochemistry and ultrastructure of polypeptide hormone-producing cells of the APUD series, and the embryologic, physiologic and pathologic implications of the concept. *J. Histochem. Cytochem.* 17:303, 1967.

2 / Hyperthyroidism

MANAGEMENT PROBLEMS

Problems experienced by the patient with hyperthyroidism include all of the features of hypermetabolism as reflected through the CNS, cardiovascular, GI, musculoskeletal, and cutaneous manifestations (Fig 2–1). Additionally, patients with Graves' disease have distinctive eye signs, such as exophthalmos, and cutaneous manifestations, such as pretibial myxedema.

The management problem for the physician caring for hyperthyroidism is to reduce the hypermetabolism of thyrotoxicosis. Longer-term goals include reducing the mass of the goiter and restoring the euthyroid state under normal pituitary control.

HYPERTHYROIDISM: HORMONES AND SYNDROMES

Hyperthyroidism has at least eight causes and may be treated by at least three major modalities—drug therapy, thyroidectomy, and radioiodine. From among the forms of hyperthyroidism listed in Table 2–1, the specific hyperthyroidism discussed in detail in this chapter is Graves' disease. The specific treatment described in detail is the role of subtotal thyroidectomy. Combined-modality treatment is the rule rather than the exception in the management of hyperthyroidism; each modality may be used as an adjunct to a primary role for one form of treatment, depending on the type of hyperthyroidism and on the circumstances of the patient.

One common cause of hyperthyroidism is iatrogenic, resulting from exogenous thyroid hormones administered in overdosage. The management of this form of hyperthyroidism is obvious. Excessive thyroid feeding will produce a syndrome with signs different from the manifestations of Graves' disease. Graves' disease is more than simple hyperthyroidism, but includes features that are not attributable to an excess of thyroid hormone. Infiltrative dermopathy and eye signs, including exophthalmos, stare, eyelid lag, and strabismus, are not due simply to excessive thyroid hormone, but to a circulating substance unique to Graves' disease called long-acting thyroid stimulator (LATS). LATS is a 7S IgG fragment of the thyroid antibody that has been postulated as etiologic in some cases of Graves' disease, but cannot be found in uniformly elevated levels in all patients who have this type

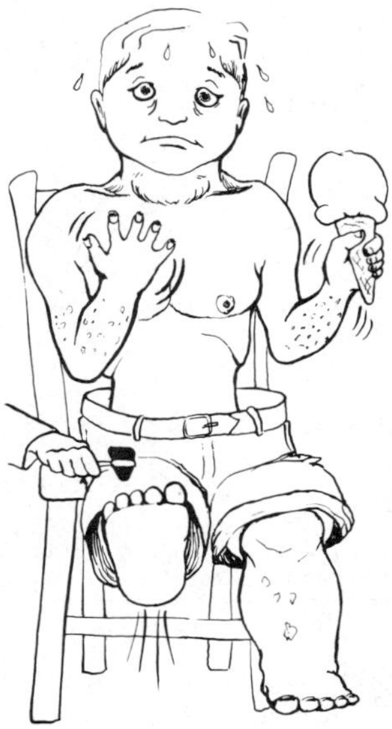

CENTRAL NERVOUS SYSTEM
- TREMOR, HYPERREFLEXIA
- SWEATING, HEAT INTOLERANCE
- SLEEPLESSNESS, PSYCHOSIS

CARDIOVASCULAR
- INCREASED STROKE VOLUME
- INCREASED CARDIAC OUTPUT
- INCREASED PULSE PRESSURE
- TACHYCARDIA, FIBRILLATION

GASTROINTESTINAL
- WEIGHT LOSS
- INCREASED APPETITE
- INCREASED INTESTINAL MOTILITY

MUSCULOSKELETAL
- WEAKNESS, FATIGUE
- PRETIBIAL MYXEDEMA
- ATROPHY OF TEMPORALIS

GENITOURINARY
- GYNECOMASTIA, INFERTILITY

EYE
- STARE, LID LAG
- EXOPHTHALMOS
- STRABISMUS

SKIN
- RASH
- HAIR AND FINGERNAIL CHANGES

THYROID
- SYMMETRIC ENLARGEMENT
- THRILL, BRUIT

Fig 2–1.—Clinical manifestations of Graves' disease.

of hyperthyroidism. LATS is implicated, however, in the ophthalmopathy of Graves' disease. The basic etiology of Graves' disease remains unknown. Control of the thyrotoxicity may not control the ophthalmopathy and other LATS-dependent features of this disorder. In most Graves' disease patients, surgical control of hyperthyroidism results in eye improvement, but this cannot be insured preoperatively.

Table 2–1 lists the other forms of hyperthyroidism, and management of several of these forms has been reviewed;[1] Graves' disease is the most common cause of hyperthyroidism and is frequently a problem for surgical management.

DIAGNOSIS

Screening for hyperthyroidism and differentiation of the forms of hyperthyroidism have been made at once simple and complex by the advent of a variety of assays for thyroid hormones and thyroid functions. Clinical signs and symptoms which suggest hyperthyroidism are confirmed by measurement of circulating thyroxine (T_4), triiodothyronine (T_3), and free thyroxine

TABLE 2–1.—DIFFERENTIAL DIAGNOSIS OF HYPERTHYROIDISM BASED ON THE PATHOPHYSIOLOGY OF THE PRIMARY PROCESS

Diffuse toxic goiter (Graves' disease)
Toxic multinodular goiter (Plummer's disease)
Toxic adenoma ("Hot nodule")
Toxic thyroiditis (Hashimoto's struma—"Hashi-tox")
Overreplacement exogenous thyroid hormone (Iatrogenic or factitial thyrotoxicosis)
Iodide therapy in endemic goiter (Jodbasedow disease)
Ectopic toxic thyroid tissue (Struma ovarii)
Paraneoplastic hyperthyroidism (Excess TSH or TSH-like paraendocrine tumors)

index (FTI). These specific thyroid hormone assays and a measure of the binding capacity for thyroid hormone have replaced a number of previous tests for thyroid function, making some of them obsolete (e.g., BMR, PBI, and BEI). Excessive circulating T_4 results in the hypermetabolic features illustrated in Figure 2–1. "T_3 toxicity" has somewhat different features: cardiovascular and emotional symptoms are prominent. T_3 toxicity is frequently a feature of Plummer's disease (see Table 2–1) and is less frequently a component of Graves' disease.

Physical examination of the thyroid gland is helpful in the differential diagnosis of hyperthyroidism. In Graves' disease, the gland is diffusely enlarged and very vascular. A bruit is often audible over the goiter. The goiter is typically uniform in its enlargement because of hyperplasia as opposed to nodule or tumor, which may give uneven enlargement. If discrete nodules are palpable, toxic multinodular goiter (Plummer's disease) or toxic adenoma may be the problem. Thyroid scanning may differentiate hyperthyroidism of these causes. In the case of toxic adenoma, the normal thyroid gland has decreased vascularity, accentuating the "hot nodule" of the adenoma on thyroid scan. If thyroid-stimulating hormone (TSH) is given, the suppressed thyroid gland surrounding the nodule may "light up" on repeated scanning. Radioimmunoassay for TSH is also available, and TSH values should be near zero in the patient with toxic adenoma or Graves' disease. If TSH is not depressed in the presence of hyperthyroidism, this finding reflects the inability of the pituitary to follow normal feedback inhibition. The diagnosis of Graves' disease is often easier to make than the differential diagnosis of some other forms of hyperthyroidism, and the patient's condition is often such that treatment is generally begun as soon as the diagnosis is confirmed.

PREOPERATIVE PREPARATION

Treatment of Graves' disease is highly individualized and depends upon the age of the patient and severity of the disease. For each of the three modalities for primary treatment of hyperthyroidism, strong advocates can be found to stress the relative advantages of their treatment method. Single-modality treatment of all forms of hyperthyroidism is risky and should be discouraged. Physicians caring for patients with thyrotoxicity must be familiar with each modality and must exercise judgment in choosing therapy combinations.

Subtotal thyroidectomy has major advantages in that its effects are immediate, with relative perioperative safety and long-term reduced risk of drug administration. Its chief advantage is that subtotal thyroidectomy can restore normal pituitary-thyroid interaction without dependence on long-term medication. Balanced against these advantages is the risk that operation alone carries in hazard to the recurrent laryngeal nerves and parathyroid glands. Each treatment modality has a risk of recurrence of hyperthyroidism and a higher probability of posttreatment hypothyroidism.

Drug treatment is essential in the perioperative management of Graves' disease. The types of drug therapy available for hyperthyroidism are listed in Table 2–2. Each of the three basic modes of antithyroid drug action is useful in the preoperative preparation of the patient with Graves' disease. The antithyroid drugs are used to decrease thyroid hormone release, production, or response. Another "drug" that may be considered in management of other forms of thyroid disease would be thyroid feeding, usually in the form of synthetic hormone administration for TSH suppression or to replace the normal thyroid hormone output. Administration of thyroid hormone has a definite role in appropriate treatment of some mass lesions or inflammatory thyroid problems (see chap. 3), but clearly would not be indicated for the patient already in a toxic state from excess circulating thyroid hormone.

The primary objective of preoperative management is to bring the patient with thyrotoxicosis to the operating room in a euthyroid state. Suppression of the overactive thyroid is not simply a desirable feature of perioperative management, but is the single most important element of a safe operation for hyperthyroidism. There is less urgency for the operative

TABLE 2–2.—TYPES OF DRUG THERAPY FOR HYPERTHYROIDISM

Decrease thyroid hormone release
Iodides (Lugol's solution)
Lithium
Decrease thyroid hormone production
Thiocyanates, perchlorates
Thionamides (PTU)
Decrease thyroid hormone response by adrenergic interference
Catecholamine depletion (reserpine, guanethidine)
β-adrenergic blockade (Propranolol)

management of hyperthyroidism than there is for preoperative control of thyrotoxicosis. Often, medical techniques of preparation of the patient may be relied upon as an option in long-term management of hyperthyroidism itself.[2] Patients may relapse into hyperthyroidism after the discontinuation of thyroid suppressive medication for as much as a year or more, or they may break through control on a fixed antithyroid medication program. Occasionally, patients have toxic reactions to the drugs used in thyroid suppression, a fact that may indicate which drugs should be employed, their sequence of administration, or the indications for earlier operation. Some series suggest that it may be possible with very prolonged antithyroid treatment to achieve remission rates in three quarters of the patients with less than 10% drug reactions and less than 5% hypothyroidism.[2]

A major advance in the safety of operative management of hyperthyroidism came with the coupling of the surgical skill of Kocher (who won the 1909 Nobel Prize for his techniques of thyroidectomy) and premedication according to Plummer, who advocated the use of Lugol's iodine preoperative preparation in 1923. The administration of iodides or lithium, as seen in Table 2–2, may be used to inhibit the release of thyroid hormone from the thyroid gland. The first of the surgically significant features of this release-inhibition is the reduction to euthyroid status; however, a second important feature is the remarkable decrease in vascularity of the goiter, as well as a shrinking of the enlarged thyroid gland. Both of these effects are useful in the preoperative preparation of the patient, since the former renders the patient metabolically manageable for the anesthetic, operation, and postoperative course, and the latter makes the operation technically easier and far less hazardous to the vital structures to be preserved in subtotal thyroidectomy.

The second class of drugs used in preoperative preparation decreases hormone production from the thyroid. These drugs act by interfering in the synthesis of thyroid hormone or by inhibition of organic incorporation of iodine. The most popular of these agents is the thionamide propylthiouracil (PTU). Agents of this class must be administered on a precise schedule, usually every eight hours, and the patient must be followed up closely for evidence of fever, joint pain, rashes, and a decrease in granulocyte count. Because of PTU's toxicity and the precision required in its administration, the patient's cooperation is necessary, and occasionally the emotional and nervous system features of Graves' disease prevent effective patient compliance.

The third class of drug therapy involves agents that decrease hormone response on the part of the target organ, regardless of circulating thyroid hormone levels. The adrenergic intermediates of hyperthyroidism can be blocked, inhibiting the effector pathway of thyrotoxicosis. Drugs that block reuptake and deplete catecholamine stores may be used for the management of thyrotoxicosis in much the same way that they are given for preoperative preparation of pheochromocytoma (see chap. 10). Direct β-adrenergic blockade with propranolol is an important advance toward rapid control of thyrotoxicity.[3] Combinations of iodide and β-blockade have been suggested[4] as the optimal preoperative preparation for patients with Graves' disease.

The selection of an agent from each class of the drugs used in preoperative preparation can be synergistically useful in combinations such as PTU, Lugol's iodine solution, and propranolol. Combinations of drugs may lessen the toxicity of a single agent and may act at different points in the synthesis and release and end-organ effect of thyroid hormone. Some combinations, as noted[4] in adding propranolol to potassium iodide, may be especially helpful in patients who have shown toxic reaction to one of the thionamides. As a substitute for operative or radioiodine ablation of the overactive thyroid gland in Graves' disease, particularly if a large goiter is present, medication has the disadvantage of a high recurrence rate of hyperthyroidism, even to prolonged drug treatment and following a prolonged period of remission. Some patients with successful drug-induced remissions in hyperthyroidism may later develop hypothyroidism. Hypothyroidism, however, is a feature of the later natural history of hyperthyroidism whether treated or not by drugs, radioiodine, or operation. This may be particularly true for patients with an inflammatory component and histologic evidence of severe thyroiditis. Although accepted as a fundamental characteristic of the later natural history of hyperthyroidism, late hypothyroidism is more frequent in the group of patients treated by radioiodine ablation.

The twin goals of preoperative drug treatment—(1) to bring the patient to the operating room in a euthyroid state; and (2) to reduce the size and vascularity of the thyroid gland—require careful consideration of the administration and sequence of the antithyroid drugs. The thyroid gland in Graves' disease is generally enlarged and very vascular, and if agents are used that inhibit hormone production (the second class listed in Table 2–2), the thyroid gland may become even more enlarged with greater blood flow. If a hormone-response-inhibitor such as propranolol is added, neither the amount of circulating hormone nor the size or blood supply of the goiter is significantly affected. Administration of iodine preoperatively for a week to ten days decreases the size of the gland, markedly diminishes its blood flow, and reduces circulating thyroid hormone. For this reason, even with the advent of newer agents, elective operation for hyperthyroidism should be immediately preceded by a course of Lugol's iodine preparation.

The importance of preoperative preparation of the hyperthyroid patient is based on the gravity and frequency of anesthetic and surgical complications that attend operating on a patient in a thyrotoxic condition. Apart from the local control of a large, very vascular goiter and the preservation of vital structures contiguous with it, the metabolic consequences of operating on the unprepared patient are serious. A dreaded complication of the manipulation of hypermetabolic patients is thyroid storm. Thyroid storm is characterized by hyperpyrexia, hyperkinesia, leukocytosis, and tachycardia in a runaway hypermetabolism, often ending in exhaustion and lethal arrhythmias, despite management with all the antithyroid drugs, added to hypothermia and paralysis on ventilator support. The extremely high mortality of this surgical complication demands that all patients operated on be prepared and rendered euthyroid before operation.

Radioiodine therapy is not often used as an adjunct to thyroid operation, but as a substitute for it. As discussed in the following chapter on thyroid nodules and cancer, the operation may frequently be adjunctive to primary radioiodine therapy. But primary radioiodine therapy for hyperthyroidism has disadvantages that accompany the considerable advantages in simplicity, cost, and relative safety, particularly in older patients. Some of the fears of radioiodine treatment that inhibit its general utility for hyperthyroidism have been largely unsubstantiated. These include the fear of carcinogenesis[5] and teratogenesis—although all final judgments on this issue require several generations for confident dismissal.

In the author's opinion, the chief drawbacks limiting the therapeutic use of radioiodine for hyperthyroidism are the prolonged induction period necessary for the gradual radioiodine control of symptoms and late hypothyroidism. Following administration of radioiodine, even if radioiodine treatment is repeated, a patient may need antithyroid drugs for several months and close monitoring for a prolonged period before tapering the medication for hyperthyroidism control. Sometimes the patient who is symptomatic or who has had a previous toxic reaction to antithyroid medication as one of the indications for radioiodine ablation remains quite uncomfortable throughout this prolonged remission induction period.

The biggest problem with radioiodine treatment of hyperthyroidism is the very high incidence of hypothyroidism. Over half of the patients who are successfully treated with radioiodine (usually those patients with smaller goiters) are clinically hypothyroid within ten years of treatment, and that number continues to increase over the ensuing decades. In a large series of well-followed patients, 70% of patients ten years after ^{131}I treatment developed clinical hypothyroidism.[6] As already mentioned, hypothyroidism may be a complication that follows subtotal thyroidectomy as well, but the hypothyroidism after operation is usually detected and managed because of its immediacy. Unlike hypothyroidism after thyroidectomy, the hypothyroidism following radioiodine treatment is insidious in onset, usually coming on long after the patient has left the primary therapist. If thyroid replacement is given in anticipation of thyroid failure following radioiodine therapy, iatrogenic recurrence of hyperthyroidism may take place.

For these reasons, a strong case may be made that the treatment of choice for Graves' disease, particularly in the younger individual in whom it is most common, is subtotal thyroidectomy in the well-prepared patient, and it is the standard against which radiation and medical management for thyroid hyperfunction are judged.

ANESTHESIA MANAGEMENT

In the well-prepared euthyroid patient, the anesthetic course for subtotal thyroidectomy should be quite simple and among the operations with the lowest morbidity. For patients with Graves' disease certain precautions should be observed to prevent problems during the period of anesthesia. Figure 2–2 illustrates the positioning of the patient with optimal cervical extension for thyroid exposure. This position, however, also places at risk the patient's eyes, which may be covered with toweling, anesthesia tubing, and other potential sources of corneal abrasion. This is particularly true for the Graves' disease patient with exophthalmos, in which case careful attention must be paid to the protection and moistening of the cornea.

Thyrotoxic patients undergoing operation require high percentages of oxygen, generally in excess of 50%, in the anesthetic mixture to satisfy the high oxidation rate in tissues. Adequate anesthesia levels must also be achieved to prevent "bucking" of the patient, particularly when the trachea is manipulated and meticulous dissection is being carried out around the

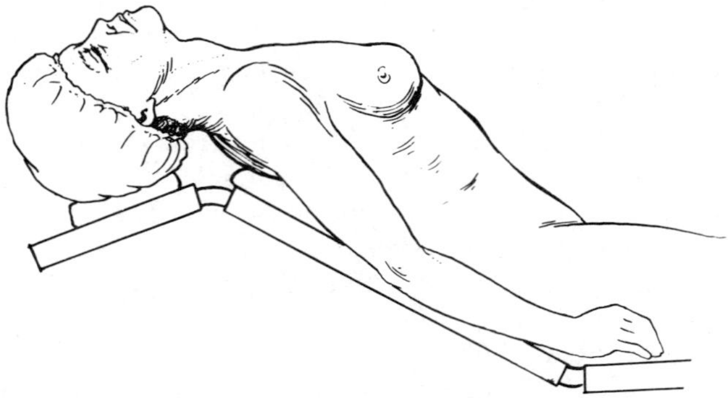

Fig 2–2.—Positioning of the patient undergoing cervical exploration for thyroid or parathyroid disease gives optimum exposure for the operation but may place the patient's corneas at risk from draping materials and anesthetic tubing, particularly if the patient has exophthalmos.

parathyroid glands and recurrent laryngeal nerves. Patient monitoring is necessary to observe evidence of cardiac arrhythmias.

The anesthesia agent of choice should be one that does not sensitize the myocardium to catecholamines or sympathomimetic drugs. Certain agents increase the circulating thyroxine, such as ether anesthesia, which also increases the salivary secretions and bronchorrhea. Thiopental sodium decreases serum thyroxine, possibly due to its thiourea nucleus,[7] and it may be the induction agent of choice for surgery in hyperthyroidism. Endotracheal intubation is mandatory, and anesthetic maintenance may best be carried out with nitrous oxide or methoxyflurane. Halothane has been reported in at least rare instances to cause ventricular fibrillation in patients with unrecognized or undertreated thyrotoxicosis, and arrhythmias may be somewhat more frequent when halothane-type anesthetic agents are used for the hyperthyroidism patient.[8]

The principal concerns in general anesthesia for hyperthyroidism are as follows: (1) the increased metabolic rate that requires the patient to have both increased minute ventilation and cardiac output, and hence reduced reserves; (2) the increased requirement for anesthetics; and (3) predisposition to cardiac arrhythmias.[9] Besides the monitoring of blood pressure and cardiac rate and rhythm, an essential feature of the operation is the monitoring of body temperature. This can be done with an indwelling temperature probe, such as an esophageal lead. A rise in temperature while the patient is under anesthesia may be an early indication of thyroid storm.

An observation of an effective technique in anesthetic management of hyperthyroidism is the availability of propranolol, and at any indication of cardiac irritability or a temperature increase, 1 mg of intravenous (IV) propranolol may be administered. This agent, even in this dosage by this route, may smooth out the anesthetic course of a patient who has received marginal preoperative preparation. It is obvious that the more desirable means of managing this complication is its prevention by a thorough preoperative preparation of the thyrotoxic patient.

OPERATIVE TECHNIQUE OF SUBTOTAL THYROIDECTOMY

The treatment of choice for hyperthyroidism in the younger individual remains subtotal thyroidectomy. Some advocates have promoted total thyroidectomy,[10,11] which obviously abolishes hyperthyroidism and reduces the potential for its recurrence to near zero. However, the author considers that total thyroidectomy is overtreatment of Graves' disease and that it eliminates the chief advantage of surgical treatment; namely, the restoration of normal pituitary-thyroid physiologic control.

Surgical management of Graves' disease swiftly accomplishes control of hyperthyroidism, may relieve mass-lesion symptoms of goiter compressing the upper airway and esophagus, and may encounter other thyroid disease such as thyroid cancer, which in the author's experience has a higher incidence than that seen in other reviews.[1] Complications of thyroid exploration should be discussed preoperatively with the patient. These include hypothyroidism, recurrence of hyperthyroidism (both of which are common to all other forms of treatment of this disorder), and hoarseness and hypocalcemia (unique to surgical therapy for hyperthyroidism). Hoarseness as a postoperative sequel may sometimes occur from the topical irritation of the endotracheal tube and the dissection around the larynx. In addition, hoarseness may frequently be due to recurrent laryngeal paresis. The hoarseness that follows operation is most often transient if the surgeon has taken care to identify and preserve the recurrent laryngeal nerves throughout their length in the dissection field. Exposing the recurrent laryngeal nerves increases the risk of transient paresis, but reduces the hazard of transection and of long-term hoarseness. Similarly, identification of the parathyroid glands and their lateral blood supply makes possible their immediate postoperative hypofunction and transient hypocalcemia, but increases the possibility of their long-term preservation. If parathyroid glands are displaced or detached in thyroid mobilization and appear to be separated from their blood supply, such a free parathyroid may be transplanted as a graft within the strap muscles by mincing it and implanting it in this source of rich blood supply.

Several modifications of surgical technique for subtotal thyroidectomy have been described. The standard technique recommends that a rim of thyroid tissue be left posteriorly along the paratracheal grooves with "no need [and it is probably unwise] to dissect and locate the recurrent nerves and the parathyroids of these patients."[12] The surgical technique for subtotal thyroidectomy that I advocate varies from this standard technique. Other available variants suggest less reduction of the thyroid with larger remnants[13] or difference in technique for the position of these thyroid remnants.[14] The operation that I prefer is to dissect both right and left thyroid lobes anatomically without entering the thyroid capsule, exposing the recurrent laryngeal nerves to the point of their entry into the larynx, and identifying parathyroid glands to avoid their inclusion in the specimen or devascularization. This technique is identical with that of total thyroidectomy until the point of locating the thyroid tissue that will be left as the thyroid remnant.

An estimated 3 to 5 gm of thyroid tissue is selected at the isthmus off the midline of the trachea, to the side of the inferior thyroid artery to be preserved. The fully mobilized goiter is dissected away from this thyroid residual, which will remain off-center along the trachea away from the paratracheal beds where the nerves and parathyroid glands have been identified. This eccentric location of the thyroid remnant obviates a prominent midline mass beneath the larynx as this residual thyroid hypertrophies in response to TSH postoperatively. To be specific in the quantity of thyroid tissue that remains, a technique in the education of surgical residents has been to use a small pathology scale in the operating room in which subtotal thyroidectomy is taking place. To improve the accuracy of estimating the amount of the residual thyroid, an identical thyroid remnant is dissected from the specimen of the resected goiter from the opposite lobe and weighed to compare it with the thyroid remnant in situ. Figure 2–3 illustrates the gross appearance of the hyperplastic thyroid gland in situ in a patient with Graves' disease, and Figure 2–4 illustrates the remnant of hyperplastic thyroid tissue that remains following subtotal thyroidectomy. In the process of cutting a comparable segment from the resected goiter specimen off the operative field, a section of the specimen is examined for evidence of any pathology beyond the expected hyperplasia. In the author's experience of 100 cases of hyperthyroidism, 9 instances of thyroid cancer were found, 8 of them by this inspection of the resected goiter in the operating room, only 1 of which had been anticipated preoperatively. If cancer is found, total thyroidectomy is completed simply by removing the thyroid remnant near the isthmus and ligating the corresponding inferior thyroid artery. The thyroid "block" has not been violated in the posterior areas of the larger mass of the thyroid lobes where nodules can be less easily felt and more easily opened (Fig 2–5).

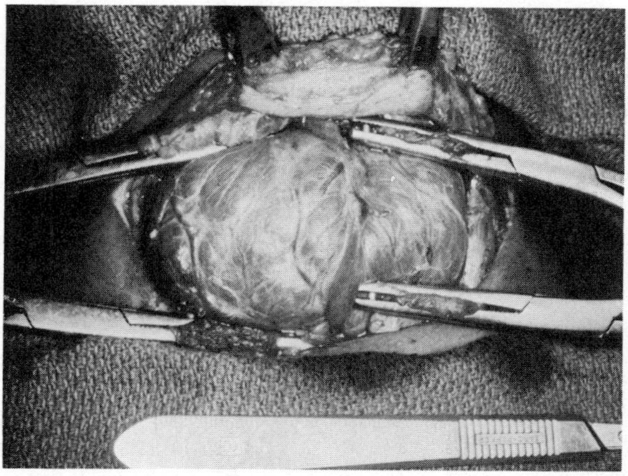

Fig 2–3.—Hyperplastic thyroid gland in situ in subtotal thyroidectomy dissection.

The advantages of this operation submitted for consideration are that the posterior dissection is cleaner and more anatomical in the critical areas in the paratracheal grooves without entering the posterior capsule. Hemostasis is easier to achieve with less risk in the case of the anterior remnant than in the hazardous clamping and suture ligature in the paratracheal regions where the bleeding, transected thyroid gland overlies the unseen

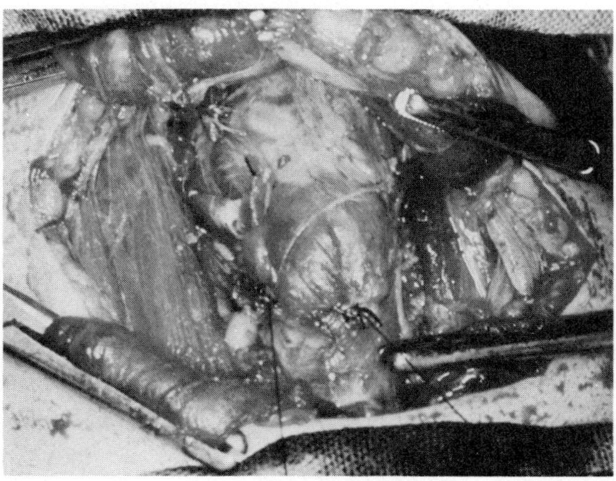

Fig 2–4.—Remnant of thyroid following subtotal thyroidectomy is, in this case, at the right of the isthmus, preserving the right inferior thyroid artery. A comparable remnant resected from the goiter specimen weighed 5 gm.

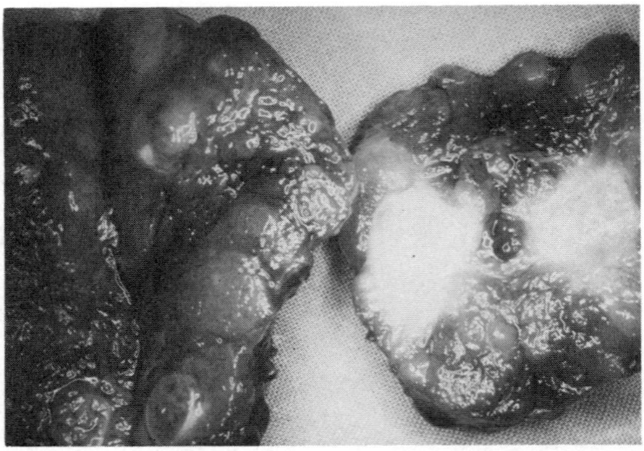

Fig 2–5.—Cut section of thyroid reveals the expected thyroid hyperplasia, but also an unexpected invasive papillary thyroid adenocarcinoma and follicular adenoma. Thyroidectomy was completed by excision of the remnant when this observation was made.

nerves and parathyroids. Delicate anatomical structures clearly seen and identified are at less risk than those which are unseen, may be aberrant, and are skirted blindly. The quantity of thyroid remnant is easier to judge at one anterior site than that located in two poorly exposed "rims." As noted, total thyroidectomy is facilitated should an unexpected finding, such as thyroid carcinoma, be encountered. Practice in this technique facilitates surgical experience of total thyroidectomy for other indications on the part of the surgical resident staff. If hyperthyroidism should recur following standard subtotal thyroidectomy, the hyperplastic remnants would be precisely where dissection would be most hazardous—on the nerves and parathyroids, almost ruling out a repeated operation and necessitating radioiodine therapy for recurrence. Postoperative thyroid scanning is more intelligible with a thyroid isthmus remnant and clear paratracheal regions.

Other options in surgical technique include the advisability of strap muscle division, particularly for a significantly enlarged goiter. A drain left in the thyroid bed for 24 hours postoperatively is a precaution in the previously hypervascular hyperthyroid patients, particularly if the preparation has been marginal. This precaution is not so much for actual drainage of any bleeding under the flaps as it is an indicator that might require opening the flap and reoperation for hemostasis—a reoperation done once in this series.

Facility in subtotal thyroidectomy is particularly useful under certain unusual circumstances, such as the hyperthyroid patient in pregnancy.[15] Reviews of large series of hyperthyroid patients treated by subtotal thyroidectomies[16] have reported generally satisfactory results from operative therapy of Graves' disease in clinics with considerable thyroid surgery experience.

POSTOPERATIVE CARE AND DRUG MANAGEMENT

To avoid constricting dressings over the airway, the wound is dressed with a folded towel, which is removed on the first postoperative day. Standard nursing care in the author's institution involves a tracheostomy set placed at the bedside and a humidifier, each of which is placed in the patient's room with or without a physician's order. If blood accumulates under the flap, a tracheostomy set is available. Never in the author's experience, nor in the institutional memory, has a tracheostomy been done for such an individual, and a simple suture removal set is adequate to open the flap to let out potentially airway-compressing blood, a simple corrective procedure that has been sufficient in the two instances of which the author is aware. The purpose of the humidifier at bedside, as far as the nursing staff can explain it, is to keep the patient awake during the postoperative night! Nose breathing is a much simpler, more efficient, and far less costly method of humidification and secretion control.

The thyroid drain is removed on the postoperative morning and the folded towel dispensed with. A postoperative calcium determination before discharge has been the practice for inpatient follow-up. Drug management has meant the conclusion of PTU and Lugol's iodine on the preoperative day, and a half dose of propranolol on the postoperative day, with discontinuation at discharge in the usual three-day hospitalization. Thyroid function studies are not monitored until the outpatient follow-up visit. Before that time, if the patient has symptomatic hypocalcemia, the symptoms rather than the values obtained in determining blood calcium are treated with oral calcium wafers. An important part of follow-up support of these persons is the psychological support, since changes are often unsettling to those patients who have preoperatively had personality disorders as a feature of their hyperthyroidism. Dr. Oliver Cope has suggested the selective use of psychotherapy in the perioperative treatment of hyperthyroidism.[17]

As part of the postoperative follow-up, a check on the thyroid function tests is usually undertaken in six weeks. For those patients who had total thyroidectomy because of a finding of coincidental cancer, thyroid replacement was begun immediately. All patients' states were immediately controlled with respect to their hyperthyroidism symptoms without antithyroid medication, and no case, to the author's knowledge, has had recurrent hyperthyroidism. The majority of patients have been euthyroid when checked in the postoperative period, and evidence of hypothyroidism is the chief indication for long-term follow-up.

FOLLOW-UP AND SPECIAL CONSIDERATIONS

Long-term follow-up of the patients in the series treated by subtotal thyroidectomy by the technique described revealed an incidence of 20% of the patients with hypothyroidism. These patients were given thyroid replacement therapy using synthetic thyroid preparations, and their circulating T_4 was assayed by the standard thyroid function tests. At one year postoperatively, patients receiving replacement therapy had their thyroid hormone and TSH levels assayed, after a period without the replacement therapy, and more than one half of them resumed thyroid replacement treatment one year after beginning this treatment. In other large series, the incidence of postoperative hypothyroidism has been reported as high as 75%,[18] beginning an average of 4.6 months after operation, with an incidence of hyperthyroidism recurrence of 1%. The higher incidence of hypothyroidism has been the stimulus behind modification of subtotal thyroidectomy techniques toward leaving larger thyroid remnants[13] with still low incidences of recurrent hyperthyroidism.

Surgical therapy remains an excellent method for the control of hyperthyroidism with acceptably low risks. The technique of subtotal thyroidectomy described in the management of hyperthyroidism should be considered one of the candidates for treatment of choice in young patients with Graves' disease. In almost all patients, combinations of the three major modalities of treatment will be employed for control of hyperthyroidism.

REFERENCES

1. Geelhoed G.W.: Hyperthyroidism; focus: surgical management. *Contemp. Surg.*12:9, 1978.
2. Slingerland D.W., Burrows B.A.: Long-term antithyroid treatment in hyperthyroidism. J.A.M.A. 242:2409, 1979.
3. Taft A.D., Irvine W.J., Sinclair I., et al.: Thyroid function after surgical treatment of thyrotoxicosis: a report of 100 cases treated with propranolol before operation. N. Engl. J. Med. 298:643, 1978.
4. Feek C.M., Sawers J.S.A., Irvine W.J., et al.: Combination of potassium iodide and propranolol in preparation of patients with Graves' disease for thyroid surgery. *N. Engl. J. Med.* 302:883, 1980.
5. Appel R., Tsangaris N., Spiegel J.: Radio-iodine treated hyperthyroidism and thyroid carcinoma. *Am. Surg.* 44:537, 1978.
6. Nofal M.M., Beierwaltes W.H., Patno M.E.: Treatment of hyperthyroidism with sodium iodide;[131] a 16-year experience. *J.A.M.A.* 197:605, 1966.

7. Oyama T.: Thyroid, in *Anesthetic Management of Endocrine Disease*. New York, Springer-Verlag New York, 1973.
8. Wolfson B., Smith K.: Cardiac arrest following minor surgery in unrecognized thyrotoxicosis: a case report. *Anesth. Analg. Curr. Res.* 46:672, 1968.
9. Bendixen H.H., Ngai S.H.: Anesthesia in thyroid surgery, Werner S.C., Ingbar S.H. (eds.): in *The Thyroid*, ed 4. Hagerstown, Md., Harper & Row, 1978, chap. 30.
10. Perzik S.L., Catz B.: The place of total thyroidectomy in the management of thyroid disease. *Surgery* 62:436, 1967.
11. Perzik S.L.: Total thyroidectomy in the management of Graves' disease: a review of 282 cases. *Am. J. Surg.* 131:284, 1976.
12. Paloyan E., Lawrence A.M.: Bilateral subtotal thyroidectomy, in *Endocrine Surgery*. Chicago, Year Book Medical Publishers, 1976, chap. 2.
13. Liechty R.D., Silverberg S.G., Hernandez J.: Limited subtotal thyroidectomy for Graves' disease. *Arch. Surg.* 116:561, 1981.
14. Bradley E.L., DiGirolamo M., Tarcan Y.: Modified subtotal thyroidectomy in the management of Graves' disease. *Surgery* 87:623, 1980.
15. Geelhoed G.W.: Surgery of the endocrine glands in pregnancy, in Weingold A.B. (ed.): *Surgical Diseases During Pregnancy*. New York, Harper & Row, 1983, chap. 8.
16. Becker W.F.: Hyperthyroidism: an experience with 245 patients treated by thyroidectomy. *J. La. State. Med. Soc.* 128:221, 1976.
17. Cope Oliver: personal communication, 1968.
18. Farnell M.B., von Heerden J.A., McConahey W.M., et al.: *Am. J. Surg.* 142:535, 1981.

3 / Thyroid Masses: Nodules, Goiter, Inflammation, and Neoplasms

MANAGEMENT PROBLEMS

Patients who have a discrete or diffuse thyroid mass may have tracheal compression, difficulty in swallowing, cosmetic deformity, and potential for thyroid cancer or fear that it may be present.

Physicians dealing with thyroid mass lesions are concerned with the differential diagnosis of thyroid masses, a nearly bewildering array of tests and diagnostic options, and judgment questions about the appropriate management with drugs, continued observation, operation, or radioiodine ablation.

THE TUMOR, ITS SYMPTOMS, AND THE DIFFERENTIAL DIAGNOSIS

In many endocrine surgical problems, subtle metabolic and endocrine effects lead the physician to infer a primary source of an excess of a normal hormone or an abnormal hormone, and then a painstaking search for localization of such a tumor. Consideration of the thyroid mass is the reverse of this usual state of affairs. Localization of the tumor is no problem, since the thyroid nodule is the presenting sign. The palpable or visible nodule leads then to the question of determining its significance. The management of the thyroid nodule is often a nonendocrine problem that happens to take place inside an endocrine gland, and the consequences for endocrinology may be limited to the fact that the endocrine function of the gland may be displaced or ablated by the presence of the mass. Consideration of thyroid mass lesions may take up a good deal of the endocrine surgeon's time, since mass lesions, even if endocrinologically insignificant, occur more frequently than thyroid hyperfunction. A number of reports are now appearing[1] regarding the question of the management of incidental thyroid masses that turn up unexpectedly in the course of cervical exploration for parathyroid disease. Incidental discoveries also take place on diagnostic studies, such as thyroid scan, in asymptomatic patients, particularly troublesome when the patient has presented with a history of radiation exposure to the head or neck. Whether thyroid mass is the presenting complaint or thyroid nodules are noted incidentally, management of these thyroid masses has endocrinologic consequences even if there is no endocrinologic abnormality at their presentation.

Thyroid mass lesions may be described as discrete—a thyroid "nodule"—or diffuse—a "goiter." Hybridization between these two types is the description of multinodular goiter. Worldwide, the incidence of goiter is 40,000/1 million. The association of goiter and iodine deficiency is well known, but is decreasing as an etiologic reason for its prevalence because of the widely available dietary iodine supplementation. There is also a remarkable gender-association, with a female-to-male sex ratio of 7.5:1. Not all of the individuals who have goiter require an operation or even any treatment, but among the large population of persons with goiter are groups at higher risk for the presence or development of potentially spreading neoplasms, of potentially manageable thyroid inflammations, or of suppressible thyroid masses; and another population more recently coming to light who have no thyroid mass palpable, but are undergoing screening for potential thyroid abnormalities because of exposure to therapeutic radiation of the head or neck. Members of each of these groups of patients are frequently reporting to physicians for examination and advice on the management of these known or potential thyroid mass lesions.

Both goiter and thyroid nodules can become massive and cause symptoms by their sheer bulk. More frequently, contemporary patients may complain of cosmetic embarrassment rather than functional impairment if the thyroid mass is superficial. Figure 3–1 shows a patient who visited the author with no personal complaint, but seeking immunizations for her child. She insisted that there were no symptoms associated with this goiter, which she did not consider abnormal, because most of her village neighbors accepted goiter as a natural feature of their appearance in her iodine-deficient part of the world. However, a much smaller thyroid mass can be symptomatic if it is interposed between the manubrium and the airway or food passages (Fig 3–2). Some unfortunate patients with undifferentiated thyroid carcinoma have rapidly expanding disease that reduces management to the prevention of strangling.

Between the extremes of masses that are asymptomatic and those that are life-threatening are the thyroid abnormalities that come to attention by causing minimal but notable symptoms. For example, some patients may complain of difficulty in breathing or of a cough when the head and neck are turned to a certain position, when they experience an impingement on the airway from an otherwise asymptomatic mass (Fig 3–3). Some patients complain of difficulty swallowing, particularly when solid food is ingested

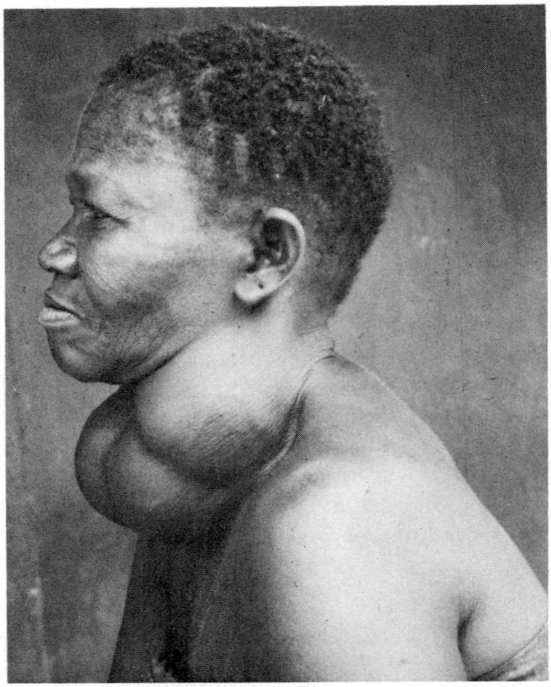

Fig 3–1.—Massive "necklace" goiter that was asymptomatic.

or when cervical extension occurs (Fig 3–4). Each of these symptoms occurs more notably in the patient who has a mass in the submanubrial space, where it may be relatively fixed anteriorly, than in a similar lesion placed in a less restrictive cervical field of the thyroid (Fig 3–5). Besides such evidence of dysfunction from space-occupying thyroid masses, the majority of patients who now appear for examination suspect or fear the presence of cancer. Management requires selectivity and judgments based on further diagnostic information.

DIAGNOSIS

History and physical examination may be sufficient evidence for a tentative diagnosis in several thyroid mass lesions. These include suppurative thyroiditis, the more common nonspecific thyroiditis, and the chronic lymphocytic infiltration from Hashimoto's thyroiditis. When standard thyroid function tests are done, results are normal in the majority of persons with thyroid mass lesions. Tests for nonspecific inflammatory response may be

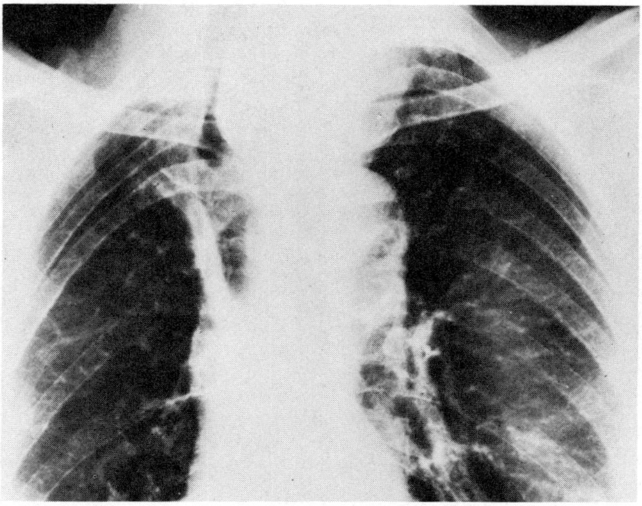

Fig 3–2.—A multinodular goiter, very symptomatic because of its deviation and compression of the airway to the extent of suffocation and syncope.

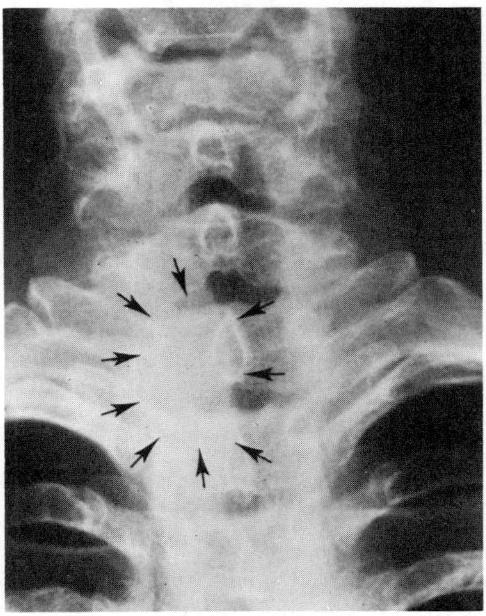

Fig 3–3.—A lesser airway compression by a thyroid nodule may be noticeable by the patient only when the head or neck assumes a specific position.

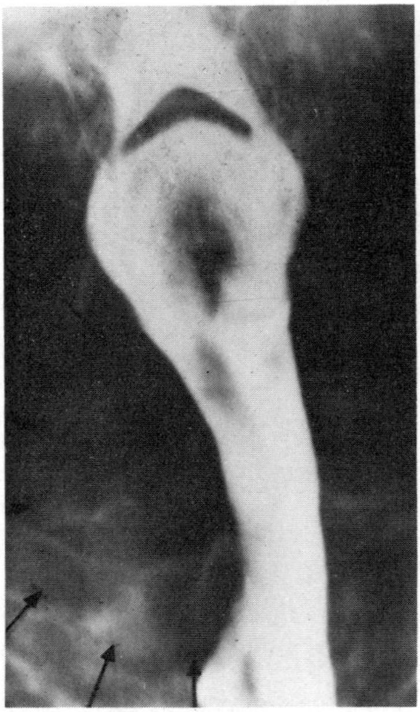
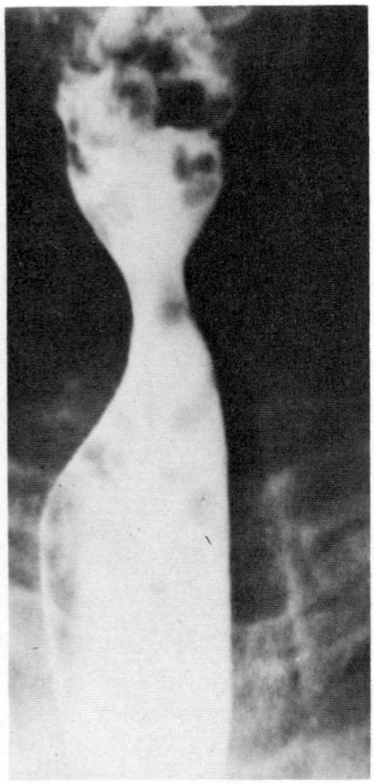

Fig 3–4 (left).—Dysphagia is reported by some patients as a feature of a thyroid nodule in posterior displacement.

Fig 3–5 (right).—Submanubrial position of this goiter means that it will give rise to symptoms earlier than a similar mass in the cervical field.

helpful in supporting the diagnosis of thyroiditis, such as sedimentation rate (SR) and white blood cell (WBC) count, and some very specific assays may be used, such as microsomal antibody determinations. In the majority of patients with tender swollen thyroids, these tests are less helpful than the clinical findings in making the diagnosis of thyroiditis. X-ray examination may be carried out to determine the indentation of the air column on tracheobronchogram (see Fig 3–3), or contrast media may be used to study displacement of cervical or thoracic organs around thyroid masses (see Fig 3–4). Rarely would arteriography be helpful, and under only specific instances would venography and venous sampling from the thyroid region be indicated, usually limited to sampling for a specific marker hormone, such as calcitonin. Medullary thyroid cancer is not a tumor of thyroid origin, but of parafollicular cells that happen to reside within the thyroid where they have migrated embryologically. Venous sampling for this tumor's specific marker may be helpful in locating disease that cannot be picked up on radioiodine scanning. Radioiodine scanning for medullary thyroid carcinoma would rely on the findings of multiple "holes" in the thyroid image by the displacement of the iodine-incorporating thyroid parenchyma. Radioiodine scanning is to no effect for diagnosis of or therapy for medullary thyroid cancer outside the thyroid gland, because the parafollicular C cells are APUD cells of different embryology and biochemistry than the thyroid parenchyma, and they do not take up or iodinate thyronine, limiting the usefulness of thyroid scanning for this specific neoplasm.

Another "shadow-producing procedure" is sonography, the use of echo devices to detect mass lesions in the region of the thyroid gland. Sonography may be helpful in determining whether a lesion is solid or cystic, and whether it changes over time by means of a relatively noninvasive test (Fig 3–6). A lesion that feels cystic on clinical examination or is consistent with a thyroid cyst by sonography might prompt needle aspiration of the fluid as the next step in management of this lesion.

Thyroid scanning is the most commonly used shadow-producing procedure and tells something of the function of the gland as well as its position. The term "cold nodule" has long been in use to describe the thyroid mass lesion that does not take up the iodine tracer as avidly as the surrounding

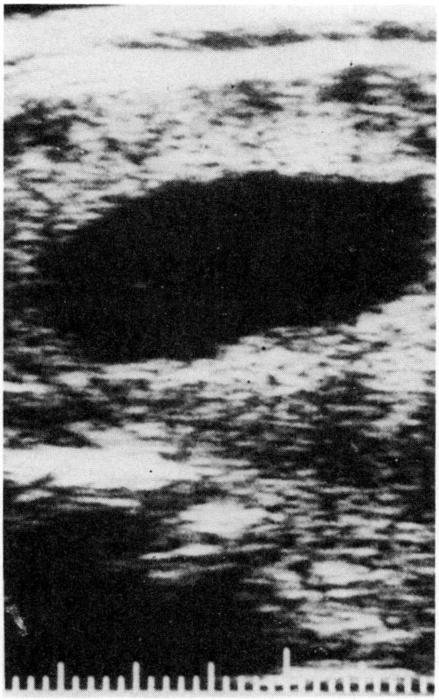

Fig 3–6.—Another "shadow-producing procedure" for discrimination of thyroid nodules is the sonogram, which can distinguish cystic from solid lesions.

tissue, giving evidence not only of its presence, but of its functional components. The "hot nodule" alluded to in chapter 2 on hyperthyroidism is often a finding accentuated because of the depression of the surrounding thyroid, since the thyroid hormone originating from the functioning hot nodule suppresses TSH, which decreases the avidity of the normal thyroid gland for iodine uptake.

These multiple, relatively noninvasive studies produce shadows, and interpretation of the shadows cast by these masses can confirm their presence, but usually does not describe their content, particularly with reference to benign or malignant character of a thyroid lesion. Physical examination is a far superior screening technique to the widespread application of these shadow-producing procedures in detecting thyroid lesions of significance. An aphorism that the author once heard attributed to Dr. George Crile was the statement, "There is no thyroid abnormality of clinical significance that cannot be palpated." With the possible exception of preclinical medullary thyroid carcinoma that can be screened in families with this disorder, I agree in principle with this statement. When evaluating thyroid abnormalities on clinical examination, I remember this general rule each time I am tempted to order one of the shadow-producing procedures in the absence of physical findings. This is particularly true in the patients who report cervical radiation exposure, and if there are no abnormalities on physical examination I resist the impulse to get multiple radiographic examinations and discourage the patient from seeking such studies.* I have operated on patients with no palpable abnormalities or radiographic evidence of lesions, directed solely by screening marker abnormalities in patients with positive family histories for medullary carcinoma of the thyroid. I have not similarly operated on random patients with no abnormality except that which appears on a radiographic image. The clinical evaluation should be the basis of prescription of therapy rather than treatment on the basis of unexplained shadows that are sometimes thought to necessitate operation. An enigmatic problem, not at all rare, is the palpation of a minimal thyroid abnormality in a patient who may report a history of thyroid radiation, and the ordering of a scan or sonogram which may show a remarkable lesion in an area of the thyroid where no abnormality is palpable. Indications for management in such a case should follow the physician's examination rather than the sometimes incidental findings on ancillary studies.

---

*One radiographic study that confirms the findings of another does not strengthen the clinical significance of these findings in the absence of symptoms or physical findings.

Isotopic scans are often thought to be mandatory preoperative studies. The thyroid scan is useful in guiding evaluation and indication for further study, but this shadow-producing procedure should not be the sole indication for operation. The information obtained by scanning depends somewhat on the isotope used, and the interpretation is coupled with the physical findings. For example, Figure 3–7,A illustrates a solitary cold nodule on thyroid scan performed with technetium on a patient who underwent exploration and was found to have a follicular adenoma of the thyroid. Figure 3–7,B illustrates a thyroid scan of an individual of the same age in whom multiple cold nodules were seen on isotopic scan. The patient was thought to have a solitary thyroid nodule by physical examination, but the multinodularity of his gland was noted, and an assumption was made that this represented a multinodular goiter. Over the ensuing follow-up, the nodules have regressed.

A technique that is becoming more widespread and is quite helpful in determining the nature of thyroid nodules short of exploration is the use of needle biopsy—and, more recently, fine-needle aspiration for cytologic studies. A dominant solitary mass in the thyroid can be aspirated with a fine needle, and the less cohesive cells of the mass when aspirated into the needle may be displayed on a microscopic slide and stained for cytologic examination. This is helpful in several kinds of thyroid problems. Some patients may be excluded from further invasive study by aspiration of inflammatory cells, confirming the diagnosis of thyroiditis. Occasionally, needle aspiration encounters a cyst that can be evacuated. On rare occasions, the author has seen lesions that presented as thyroid masses, which on aspiration revealed metastatic carcinoma from previously unsuspected sites of origin. (One recent solitary thyroid nodule was correctly diagnosed by aspiration cytology as hypernephroma, and attention was directed from the thyroid gland to the primary source.) Needle aspiration is often helpful in sparing patients further consideration of thyroid exploration, and therapy may be directed by the specific diagnoses that can sometimes be made cytologically.

Aspiration cytology results in the majority of thyroid nodules, however, may be equivocal or unhelpful with the important distinction between benign and malignant. Rarely can one make a diagnosis of endocrine organ cancer by cytologic criteria. Even under histologic examination, the character of the cells and their pattern is less often significant than is their invasion of surrounding structures for the determination of malignancy. This is not possible typically on cytologic aspiration, and a frequent diagnosis from the aspiration of a dominant thyroid nodule would be "follicular neoplasm." Such a diagnosis does not prescribe further operation, since the

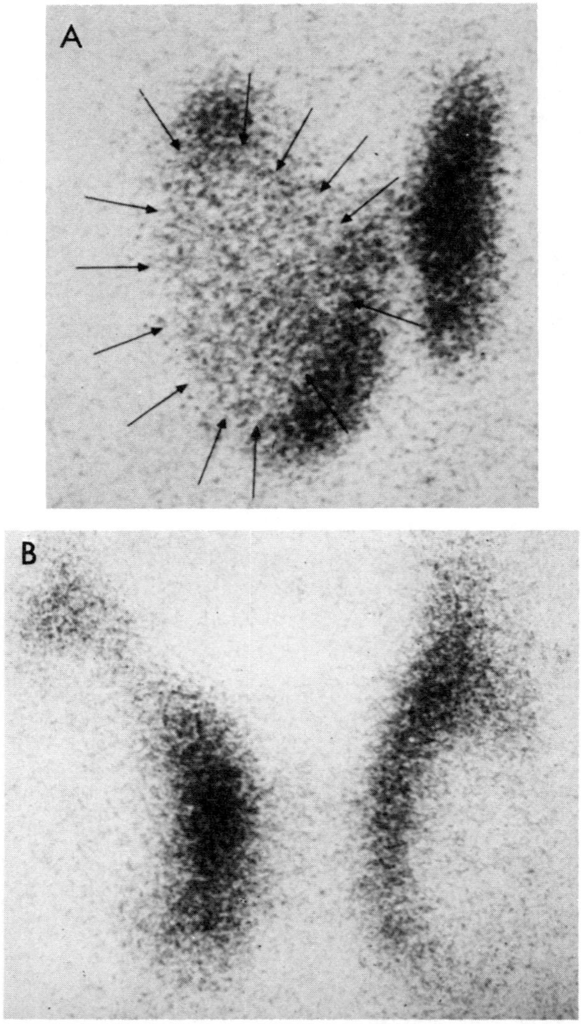

Fig 3–7.—A, solitary "cold nodule" on thyroid scan; iodine, technetium, or other tracers are employed. **B,** multiple "cold nodules" seen on isotopic scan of another patient's thyroid gland.

essential distinction would be between a follicular adenoma and carcinoma. The value of this information is limited, therefore, and further evidence is required on which to base a further course of observation or operation.

In general, thyroid cysts are managed by aspiration of the fluid content. If the mass is completely aspirated, the patient is rescheduled for a follow-up visit, and aspiration may be repeated if the cyst fluid reaccumulates. If a residual mass is present, the mass after fluid aspiration is dealt with as a solitary thyroid nodule. Frequently a fine needle can be introduced into the mass, and aspiration cytology obtained on the cells obtained, although it is not generally the author's practice to send cyst fluid for cytologic evaluation because of the low yield of evaluable cells. The patient who reports previous head and neck irradiation is examined carefully for evidence of palpable thyroid abnormality. In the absence of clinical findings, the patient is scheduled for semiannual thyroid examinations, with a note appended to his chart that at any physical examination special attention should be directed to the thyroid examination. The awareness of the patient is frequently sensitization enough for the examining physician. Routine or interval thyroid scans are not ordered; if the patient returns for a repeated evaluation carrying a thyroid scan ordered by another physician whom he had told about his thyroid radiation (a history frequently difficult to confirm with specific dosages to the unprotected thyroid), the physical examination is still relied upon more heavily than any abnormality in the thyroid image. However, if a nonpalpable thyroid defect is seen on the scan, aspiration cytology is carried out in this area. In observing the results of thyroid operations performed solely on the basis of scan information obtained from patients who reported thyroid radiation, no instance of significant thyroid pathology that would ordinarily require surgical treatment has been encountered in a ten-year period at one university hospital.

PREOPERATIVE PREPARATION

For the patient with no evidence of thyroid hyperfunction, preoperative preparation is essentially limited to the routine preanesthetic insurance of normal cardiopulmonary and renal status. One of the elements of preoperative preparation that may be used to occasionally exclude operation is a trial of thyroid hormone administration to suppress TSH. There are strong advocates for this procedure, and equally strong detractors who say that at best it may delay decision without primarily affecting any basic changes. As an arbitrary compromise, thyroid suppression is employed for multinodular glands and generally not used for solitary nodules.

Some solitary nodules in young women are reported as very rapidly enlarging, usually a sign of an adenoma with hemorrhage and liquefaction. These patients may express symptoms of this rather quickly arising mass, and occasionally therapeutic needle aspiration may relieve the symptoms. If the mass does not resolve or reaccumulates, thyroid exploration is generally advised for control of such masses.

In the event that needle aspiration can enable one to confidently predict that a thyroid cancer will be encountered (and this confidence is generally a product of considerable experience in the cytologic evaluation of thyroid nodules, with a learning curve surpassing several hundred patients), preparations can be made for a total thyroidectomy. The patient may be informed that thyroid exploration will involve careful intraoperative examination of the entire thyroid gland because of the frequent multicentricity of disease, even in the absence of preoperative palpation, scanning, or sonographic evidence of more than one lesion. The primary suspicious lesion is then going to be passed to the pathologist along with the lobe surrounding it, and based on results of frozen section examination and operative findings, a decision will be made as to the extent of the thyroidectomy. Generally speaking, patients who have had a preoperative diagnosis of carcinoma on the basis of cytology are informed that if this finding is confirmed and the carcinoma is found to be invasive through the capsule surrounding the primary nodule, a total thyroidectomy will be carried out depending on the cell type and aggressive appearance reported by the pathologist. The risks of total thyroidectomy are explained to each patient undergoing exploration, and consent for this procedure obtained even if the likelihood of total thyroidectomy is not very high. Thyroid exploration for mass lesion is rarely urgent, and it may be scheduled electively at the patient's convenience without the fixed schedule imposed by careful preparation of preoperative hyperthyroid patients.

An important exception, which is infrequently encountered but is an indication of major importance from the yield in cytologic preoperative study, is the report of medullary thyroid carcinoma on fine-needle aspiration. If this report is obtained, the patient is screened preoperatively for any evidence of catecholamine hypersecretion to rule out pheochromocytoma before any consideration of an elective cervical operation.

In addition, a baseline plasma calcitonin determination is made and urinary calcitonin excretion collected. The results are not awaited before proceeding with therapy, but are helpful later in establishing a baseline preoperative value for postoperative calcitonin follow-up as a marker.

ANESTHESIA MANAGEMENT

General considerations for anesthesia for the patient with a thyroid mass are no different from the evaluation of the patient's anesthesia risk factors for undergoing any elective operation. Specific problems, however, involve the airway. Mechanical problems can be present from a thyroid mass that indents or deviates the trachea, making endotracheal intubation somewhat difficult. One of the more severe respiratory obstructions that may be encountered after the resection of the thyroid mass may be tracheomalacia from prolonged impingement on the cartilaginous rings of the trachea. This rare lesion may not be appreciated until after the removal of the thyroid mass and the structural failure of the trachea is seen. Prolonged intubation may be required, and external support of the trachea secured by synthetic tracheal rings sewn into position. Such management was employed for a patient (see Fig 3–2) who had tracheomalacia as his chief postoperative problem following the removal of a very large recurrent goiter that had been present for over 30 years.

Airway management mandates the secure placement of an endotracheal tube for the dissection around the upper airway. Bleeding may occur under the flaps after closure and before extubation, and it is important for the anesthesiologist to closely observe the patient in the few minutes after extubation to insure that the patient is breathing easily without the tube in place. Extubation may be done with a laryngoscope to examine the motion of both cords as the patient coughs on reawakening. Stridor at this point following operation may suggest hypofunction of at least one vocal cord. If both vocal cords are not moving, consideration of reintubation is necessary as the patient awakens further.

In addition to airway compromise from hemorrhage, which may develop under the closed cervical flaps, a more subtle form of airway compromise is seen with pneumothorax.[2] Tension pneumothorax may result from dissection that enters the mediastinum or lateral inferior cervical field, and if the patient should experience this form of respiratory distress with an intubated airway under good control, the pneumothorax should be treated simultaneously with its diagnosis. This can be carried out with the patient still obscured by the operating field drapes by inserting a needle on a large-caliber syringe into each pleural space. The plunger will be pushed from the barrel on the affected side, simultaneously affecting diagnosis and treatment. For longer follow-up, a chest tube can be placed if there is continued accumulation of air in the chest.

OPERATIVE MANAGEMENT

The patient positioning for thyroid operations for mass lesions is the same as that illustrated for thyroid hyperfunction (see Fig 2–2). If the operation is to be limited to the thyroid and the anterior cervical field, skin preparation and draping are carried out from the chin to the mid-chest. For operations in which an extension of the thyroidectomy is expected to lateral neck dissections, such as for medullary thyroid carcinoma, an appropriately larger field is prepared and draped.

For most instances of large thyroid mass, the strap muscles might be divided, particularly on the side of the lesion, to facilitate adequate exposure and careful dissection and preservation of recurrent laryngeal nerve and parathyroids on the affected side. A careful search for other foci in the opposite lobe of the thyroid is undertaken as the pathologist examines the specimen. The report of an invasive thyroid carcinoma may indicate the completion of the thyroidectomy, employing techniques similar to the description of subtotal thyroidectomy, except that no thyroid remnant is left behind.

Total thyroidectomy is preferred for the treatment of invasive thyroid carcinoma for several reasons. A thyroid remnant is not sought to support thyroid function, since it is unnecessary. The patient will receive thyroid replacement therapy in any event, regardless of the extent of the dissection, in order to suppress TSH to prevent the stimulation of any residual disease. A second major reason is that total thyroidectomy facilitates thyroid scanning. If any residual disease remains within the lymph nodes or other fields of the neck that could not be appreciated at the time of the operation, but does take up the radioiodine on diagnostic scanning, this minimal disease would not be appreciated if any considerable portion of the thyroid were present as an "iodine sink" capturing most of the iodine, reducing the sensitivity of the diagnostic scan. A third reason is that thyroidectomy becomes an adjunctive surgical technique, facilitating radioiodine therapy. By ablating the thyroid gland, the iodine sink is eliminated, thereby facilitating delivery of the radioiodine to microscopic metastatic foci, possibly with a reduced dose of radioiodine. In follow-up, repeated diagnostic scanning may indicate recurrence or further spread of the disease, not likely to be noted if any considerable portion of the thyroid remains following near-total or subtotal thyroidectomy. Total thyroidectomy is nearly as safe as any of its modifications in the hands of an experienced surgical team. This is not to deny the increased risk of transient hypocalcemia or the possibility of an increased risk of dysfunction of the recurrent laryngeal nerves in their dissection and exposure. But the potential for long-term hoarseness or hypocalcemia will not be appreciably different for the patient treated by total thyroidectomy or near-total modifications.

There are few indications for radical neck dissection along with primary thyroid exploration, unless specific cell type and malignant behavior are known or strongly suspected at the time of the operation. In the course of the thyroid dissection, the central compartment of the neck is exposed, and a careful check is made for the lymph nodes visible within this central cervical field. Indication for radical neck dissection should follow the behavior of the disease, and further diagnostic information from scanning or from fine-needle aspiration of any palpable lateral neck masses. Radical neck dissection is reserved, in the author's experience, for medullary thyroid carcinoma and for highly aggressive thyroid malignant cell types, already demonstrably metastasized. For most thyroid neoplasms, radical neck dissection is a "punishment that does not fit the crime." The benefit of extirpation of these malignant cells comes at a high risk of dysfunction, with the loss of the spinal accessory nerve and other sequelae of the neck dissection that are more acceptable for epidermoid lesions of the head and neck, which do not have another option of therapy as effective as radioiodine is for functioning thyroid metastases.

The range of thyroid operations can be illustrated by Figure 3–8, depicting a predictably benign follicular adenoma of the thyroid gland, which was removed with a subtotal lobectomy on the affected side. Figure 3–9 illustrates the cervical field following radical thyroidectomy with bilateral neck dissection for a very extensive medullary thyroid carcinoma that had evolved from a very small primary thyroid neoplasm to involve all the lymph nodes examined in the neck dissection specimens.

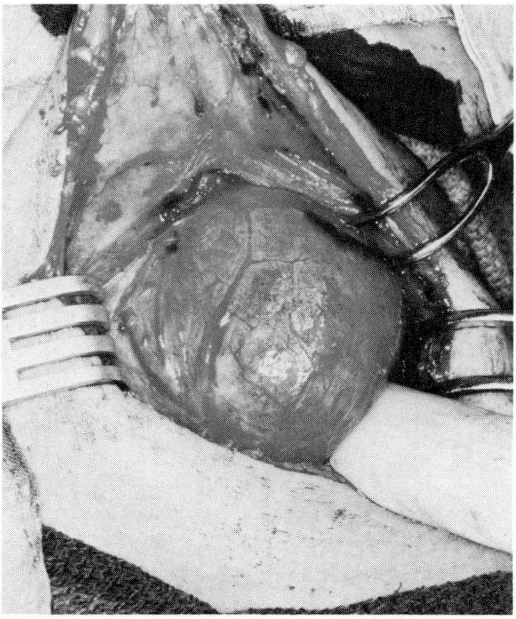

Fig 3–8.—Some solitary thyroid nodules may be predictably benign, but are removed because of the cosmetic or functional embarrassment caused by their mass—as in the case of this follicular adenoma, removed by limited resection.

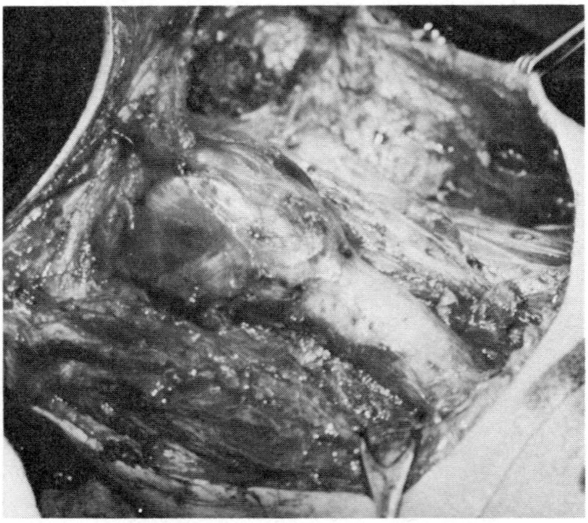

Fig 3–9.—The other extreme of the cervical exploration—in this instance for medullary thyroid carcinoma known preoperatively to have metastasized to bilateral cervical nodes—showing radical thyroidectomy with simultaneous neck dissection.

POSTOPERATIVE CARE AND MANAGEMENT

Following operation for a thyroid mass, the patient may have normal thyroid function if subtotal thyroidectomy or less dissection has been performed. For some lesions, including most of the malignant thyroid nodules, thyroid replacement therapy is suggested for suppression of TSH. Thyroid replacement is mandatory for patients who have undergone total thyroidectomy. However, this thyroid replacement is not started immediately, but a period of time is allowed to elapse, usually about six weeks from thyroidectomy, until hypothyroidism begins to become apparent. This allows the build-up of TSH and facilitates the postoperative diagnostic scanning, it also aids in the incorporation of therapeutic radioiodine for those patients for whom it is indicated. If some patients are thought to have indications for earlier treatment or are very symptomatic with early hypothyroidism, exogenous TSH can be administered to facilitate incorporation of the radioiodine.

The majority of patients who undergo operative extirpation of mass lesions have a simple operation and an uneventful postoperative course. The majority of those patients with thyroid nodules are reported to have follicular adenoma or some variation of a benign lesion. For proved invasive thyroid cancers, some investigators advocate use of a protocol to follow up such patients with diagnostic scanning and radioiodine administration for therapeutic purposes (Table 3–1). Depending upon the cell type and behavior of the neoplasm demonstrated in the patient's clinical course, a modification of this protocol is followed for patients with frankly invasive thyroid cancer.

FOLLOW-UP AND SPECIAL CONSIDERATIONS

For some patients with benign adenomas or inflammatory thyroid disease, follow-up therapy may employ thyroid suppression or anti-inflammatory drug treatment. For thyroid cancer, serum thyroglobulin may be a useful follow-up marker. For patients with specific forms of thyroid malignant disease, such as medullary thyroid carcinoma, the follow-up may use the hormone marker of these parafollicular APUD cells in the form of calcitonin in urine and serum, particularly following calcium or pentagastrin stimulation. Venous sampling can also locate recurrent disease in the absence of ability to detect it on scan or in the absence of palpable and aspirable lesions. Patients with this form of APUD malignancy have responded to reoperation and reduction of tumor burden. Streptozocin may be effective for this malignant disease, and other antimetabolite drugs may be used for thyroid malignancy in addition to the radioiodine that is specific for those functioning thyroid cancers that incorporate it. The thyroid hormone can be used as a marker for the functioning thyroid carcinoma that has metastasized; also, the assay of serum thyroid hormone levels helps in the management of replacement therapy.

TABLE 3–1.—PATIENT MANAGEMENT FLOW SHEET

Thyroid cancer on frozen section, then
1. Operation—(near) total thyroidectomy
2. Wait six weeks Serum T_4 and TSH
3. Scan neck and total body ^{131}I
4. RAI Rx if tissue uptake is positive —Low-iodine diet and diuretics
5. Suppress with L-thyroxine
6. One year later —Switch to T_3
7. Wait three weeks —Serum T_4 and TSH —Rescan with ^{131}I
8. Follow serum T_G —Re-treat patient with ^{131}I if scan is positive

Although the majority of thyroid masses are endocrinologically insignificant, management of thyroid mass lesions constitutes a significant proportion of the endocrine surgeon's attention. The best indicator of diagnosis and the most reliable predictor of those patients who could benefit from operation is a careful physical examination. Some discrimination can be achieved with tests that produce shadows, which can define the position, number, and nature of the masses, but cannot distinguish generally between the benign and malignant ones. Aspiration cytology is useful when a positive diagnosis of specific cell types can be made in predicting malignancy, but is less useful as an indicator of benign nodules. Thyroid exploration removes mass lesions that are benign, and helps to control thyroid malignancy as an adjunct to radioiodine for functioning thyroid carcinoma and as an adjunct to chemotherapy by tumor reduction for medullary thyroid carcinoma.

REFERENCES

1. Al-Jurf A., Esselstyn C.B., Crile G. Jr.: Thyroid lesions in patients with hyperparathyroidism. *Int. Surg.* 64:33, 1979.
2. Bendixen H.H., Ngai S.H.: Anesthesia in thyroid surgery, in Werner S.C., Ingbar S.H. (eds.): *The Thyroid,* ed 4. Hagerstown, Md., Harper & Row, 1978, chap. 30.

4 / Hyperparathyroidism

MANAGEMENT PROBLEMS

Patients with hyperparathyroidism may be asymptomatic with no complaints except for an incidental screening abnormality on multiphasic biochemical testing. However, in many cases the patients experience problems from this hypercalcemia that may take the form of thirst, weight loss, renal colic, polyuria, bone and joint pains, pathologic fractures, abdominal pain, heart block, hypertension, weakness, headache, confusion, lethargy, and, ultimately, coma.

The management problem for the endocrine surgeon is to screen and interpret hypercalcemia and differentiate the hypercalcemia of hyperparathyroidism. Primary hyperparathyroidism yields effectively to surgical therapy when the exploration uncovers the source of the parathormone excess, and restores the patient to normocalcemic parathyroid function. Difficult problems arise with persistent or recurrent hyperparathyroidism, and the obverse may also result when hypoparathyroidism follows extirpation of the functioning parathyroid tissue. Localization becomes a problem of major importance when dealing with the small and frequently aberrant parathyroid that is at fault for the production of hyperparathyroidism.

HYPERPARATHYROIDISM: A CORRECTABLE HYPERCALCEMIA

Hypercalcemia is not rare, and hyperparathyroidism is not its only, or even its leading, cause. Malignancy in some nonparathyroid organ is the most frequent source of hypercalcemia, caused by demineralization of bone from metastases. Particularly if hypercalcemia is of abrupt onset, and especially if there are symptoms that may not be referable to hyperparathyroidism in the effect of hypercalcemia, malignant disease must be ruled out. This is done by checking the other data in the multiphasic screening that diagnosed the hypercalcemia. If there are no abnormalities in the biochemistry, a chest x-ray, abdominal x-ray, and intravenous pyelogram (IVP) may be helpful in uncovering abnormalities that were not apparent on physical examination.

Other endocrine disease may cause hypercalcemia, such as hyperthyroidism. Some patients take medications that are prescribed or self-administered, such as thiazide diuretics, vitamin D, or milk and antacids for treatment of peptic ulcer disease. Sarcoidosis, multiple myeloma, and some rare malignant tumors may cause hypercalcemia as well, some of the latter because of the secretion of a paracrine parathormone-like substance.

In some contexts, however, malignant disease is unlikely, and hyperparathyroidism becomes the most common source of the hypercalcemia. Such conditions include hypercalcemia of long standing at serum calcium levels that are not severely elevated and in patients who have minimal or no symptoms referable to any specific organ system. Some of these patients have hyperparathyroidism that is stimulated by some other primary organ deficit; for example, chronic renal failure can give rise to high serum phosphorus and chronically low ionized calcium levels, stimulating the parathyroid glands to become hyperplastic and resulting in the syndrome of secondary hyperparathyroidism. Under some circumstances, patients with renal failure and established secondary hyperparathyroidism may have the hyperplastic glands switch to autonomous hyperfunction, a condition known as tertiary hyperparathyroidism. Those patients with hyperparathyroidism that appears to be parathyroid in origin primarily are far more common than was thought just a decade before widespread use of the serum AutoAnalyzer, and hyperparathyroidism may now be ranked as one of the most common endocrinologic abnormalities. If the autonomous hyperfunction of one or more parathyroid glands is brought under control by the excision of the abnormal tissue, and successful normal function resumes of the parathyroid tissue that remains, hyperparathyroidism is an eminently curable form of hypercalcemia. Hyperparathyroidism is well worth searching for, moreover, because the complications of long-standing hypercalcemia can be prevented by means of this operation on patients early in their course before renal, skeletal, ocular, or neurologic complications ensue.

DIAGNOSIS

The diagnosis of hypercalcemia requires a reliable and repeated indication of an elevated level of serum calcium. If this serum calcium is elevated and the serum phosphate appears to be depressed, a further determination may be made of the serum chloride. If the chloride-to-phosphate ratio is greater than 33 in a patient with hypercalcemia, the diagnosis of primary hyperparathyroidism is very likely.[1] It is important to point out, however, that these biochemical and more subtle indicators of hyperparathyroidism apply in the "virginal patient"—one not taking medications such as thiazide diuretics or vitamin D. At least one particularly difficult diagnostic dilemma in the author's experience was resolved with the hydrocortisone suppression test, in which the serum calcium level decreased after one week of steroid treatment, making the diagnosis of hyperparathyroidism very unlikely.[2]

The availability of immunoassays for serum parathyroid hormone and the ability to test for ionized serum calcium both are helpful in equivocal cases, but are not necessary in all patients with hyperparathyroidism. Often, specialized assays require an extended period of time for their determination and may vary in their reliability. However, in a patient with prolonged low levels of hypercalcemia, with no provable malignant source elsewhere, and with a compatible biochemical pattern, hyperparathyroidism is the convincing diagnosis. Most of the patients now referred for hyperparathyroidism have usually had a parathormone value obtained as well as biochemical data showing hypercalcemia of at least 11.0 mg/dl on several occasions. It is important to have this conviction on the basis of the usual clinical and biochemical evidence, rather than waiving some of the contrary classic criteria in favor of isolated more sophisticated assays. Patients with hyperparathyroidism are not selected for operation on the basis of a number or a nomogram, but these frequently asymptomatic patients are convinced that they might benefit from operation only by a thoroughly convinced surgeon who knows that he will be staking on this diagnosis his professional acumen and perhaps many tedious hours to confirm and correct the problem at the initial thorough exploration.

PREOPERATIVE PREPARATION

Preoperative preparation is minimal in the patient who is asymptomatic or who has classic hyperparathyroidism. This is not the case for the atypical individual with hyperparathyroidism of the severe disorder known as "parathyroid poisoning."[3] This form of severe hypercalcemia is a life-threatening crisis in which GI and cardiovascular symptoms precede stupor and coma. Many of the patients with this parathyroid poisoning have large tumors that are sometimes even palpable on physical examination.[4] The patient who presents in this form of hypercalcemia crisis is one of the rare indications for an emergency parathyroidectomy. However, this should only be undertaken when the diagnosis is certain and the patient optimally prepared for the operating room and anesthetic. The steps taken in immediately resuscitating the individual include hydration and diuresis, IV phosphate infusion, and corticosteroid administration. The mainstay of treatment for parathyroid crisis is the infusion of large volumes of IV fluids with furosemide treatment. This diuretic and hydration method is effective in reducing toxic levels of hypercalcemia in all but the rare patient who might be considered a candidate for urgent parathyroidectomy. Other drugs are less useful in the management of hypercalcemia from hyperparathyroidism than they are in reducing hypercalcemia of malignancy. Drugs that are available for the management of hypercalcemic crisis include calcitonin, which is commercially available as a salmon calcitonin preparation. It has a good effect in reducing serum calcium without the toxicities of phosphate infusion and the antimetabolite drug, Mithramycin, and can be given to the patient with impaired renal function and cardiac effects, typical results of the parathyroid poisoning. Mithramycin is one further step in reducing serum calcium, and is usually given IV as a single dose

If, during the steps in the hypercalcemic management, an x-ray film can be obtained of the skull or hands that shows subperiosteal bone resorption, the patient can be confidently taken to the operating room for an urgent parathyroidectomy.[5]

The firm conviction of the diagnosis of hyperparathyroidism is all the localization necessary before primary operative exploration. The operation itself is the most effective and safest means of localization of parathyroid tissue, both normal and abnormal. There are some suggestions that gray-scale sonography and CAT scanning may be useful adjuncts in the preoperative preparation of the patient, but are often used to support a somewhat tentative diagnosis on the basis of clinical and biochemical evidence. Furthermore, it is less helpful to have a preoperative localization of a tumor in hyperparathyroidism that has not been previously operated upon, because the intent of the operation is to confirm the presence and identify the position of all parathyroid tissue, not just direct attention to a parathyroid tumor, and the noninvasive radiographic tests do not show normal parathyroid tissue.

ANESTHESIA MANAGEMENT

The anesthesiologist's evaluation will include evidence of renal damage, mental depression or confusion, muscle hypotonia, ECG evidence of hypercalcemia (short QT intervals and nearly absent ST segments), and other evidence of muscle weakness, vomiting, and electrolyte imbalance.[6] Evidence of any of these features on preoperative evaluation may lead to an intensification of the steps outlined above to reduce serum calcium. However, the management of the anesthetic course will be modified to minimize the dose of muscle relaxants in patients who are hypotonic. Care must be exercised in padding of pressure points and areas of superficial nerves in these patients, since the operation and anesthetic course may be prolonged, and the patient may be immobilized for an extended period in cervical hyperextension.

OPERATIVE TECHNIQUE

The author believes that every parathyroid exploration ought to be undertaken as a large operation that may be prolonged, and conditions should be arranged as close to ideal as possible. It is far better to begin the operation with a careful, wide-field preparation, a large cervical incision, strap muscle division, a fresh surgical team, and to be surprised at the ease with which the operation is carried out, than to be humbled by the mushrooming difficulty of the procedure that starts with inadequate preparation and abuts deadlines and other responsibilities (Table 4–1).

The best chance the patient has to be relieved of hyperparathyroidism falls to the surgeon who first explores the neck. If conviction is the keynote of the decision to operate, concentration is the keynote of the operation. The operation is undertaken deliberately and patiently, with attention focused on the usual and ectopic sites of parathyroid glands. It is more frequently a disappointment to the author to encounter a large parathyroid adenoma immediately, since this makes the search for the normal parathyroid glands more tedious. The major part of the operation does not come with the encounter of the principal pathology, but with the completion of the search for at least four parathyroid foci. The danger in an early encounter with a parathyroid adenoma is that the operation may be terminated as an anticlimax to this adenoma discovery. If the other glands are not en-

TABLE 4–1.—CONVICTION OF DIAGNOSIS: HYPERPARATHYROIDISM

Careful positioning of patient with cervical hyperextension
Fresh surgical team with no deadline times
OR table at correct height, surgeons and assistants comfortable
Collar incision at least 10 cm
Rubberband suspension of superior cervical flap
Division of strap muscles
First assistant retracting thyroid with gauze-wrapped finger
Second assistant retracting lateral incision with Green retractor
Circulating nurse insuring direction of light
Preparation of 4 specimen labels, containers, and thyroid "map"
Pathologist on call, aware of forthcoming specimens
Confirmation of 4 parathyroid glands before closure

countered, the adenoma is indistinguishable from three unseen, similarly hyperplastic, glands. If an adenoma is encountered and there is a normal parathyroid gland on one side of the neck, being content with this information may cause one to overlook multiglandular disease, which occurs in approximately 5% of patients, despite the findings of one large and one normal parathyroid gland (Fig 4–1).

The identification and confirmation of at least four parathyroid glands is the stated objective of parathyroid exploration. Only after all four glands are identified are normal glands biopsied or suspicious glands removed. The pathologist should be called only once for confirmation of these tissues, which are carefully labeled as they are biopsied and placed in containers specifically labeled as to their origin and right or left, superior or inferior positions (Fig 4–2). The technique of biopsy of the normal parathyroid glands advocated by the author has been previously described,[7] involving application of a small metallic ligating clip on the side opposite the vascular hilum, exercising care not to infarct or avulse the parathyroid gland intended for preservation. Should the pathologist report failure to confirm parathyroid tissue in one of the specific sites that has been labeled on the four specimens he has received, a careful search can be made in the region in question, with the metallic clip as a marker for the previous biopsy. At the time of the previous description of this biopsy technique, the metallic

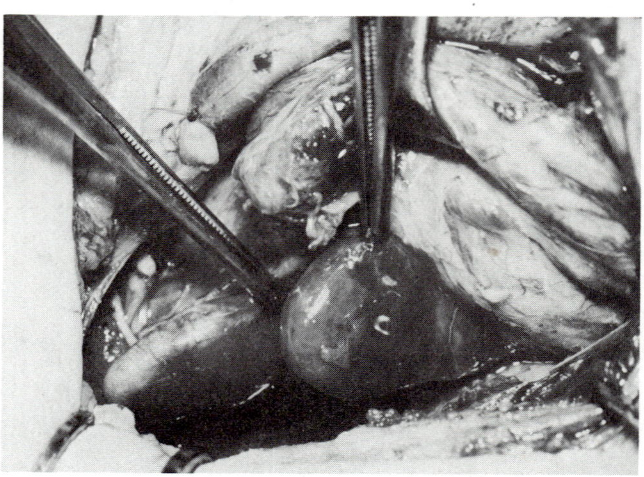

Fig 4–1.—It is possible to encounter multiple parathyroid adenomas, so that identification of one putative enlarged gland and one normal parathyroid does not complete the operation.

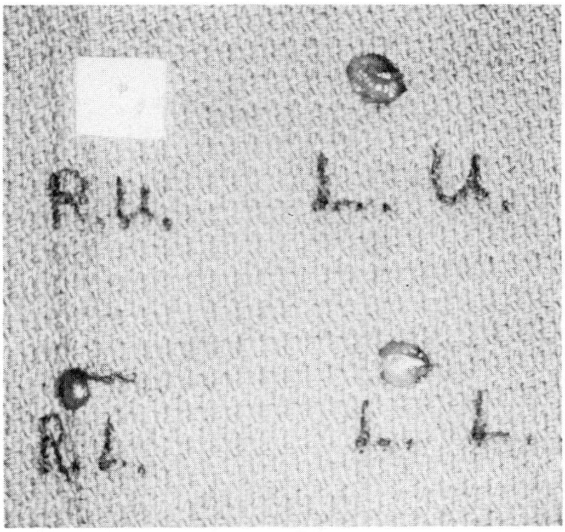

Fig 4–2.—The pathologist should be called only once to confirm on frozen section all four glands the surgeon has grossly identified. Three glands that appear normal are biopsied and the suspicious gland excised after all four are discovered.

clips were helpful markers for reexploration or for radiography by arteriographic or venographic techniques. Since that description, the use of CT scanning has made them less beneficial and more hazardous, and the author is presently using[8] a nonopaque marking clip for the same purposes—hemostasis, biopsy, and marking for later identification.

Exploration for hyperparathyroidism is very gratifying if all four glands are encountered, particularly if a parathyroid adenoma is removed (Fig 4–3). From the majority of cases that fall into this category, to get the extra percentages requires skill and patience, coupled with detailed information as to the embryology and anatomy of ectopic parathyroid locations. The search for a missing gland should proceed by deliberate plan, as methodically as the initial exploration that uncovered the first three (Table 4–2).

Particularly if the missing gland appears to be an inferior parathyroid gland, and especially if the missing gland is the suspected adenoma by pathologic confirmation of three normal parathyroids, a careful exploration of the inferior thyroid arteries' branches is in order, particularly on the side where a fourth parathyroid gland has not been reported. If any significant branches of the inferior thyroid artery are found to enter the submanubrial mediastinum, these branches are carefully followed, and gentle palpation of the submanubrial space is carried out. The thymus can be delivered with

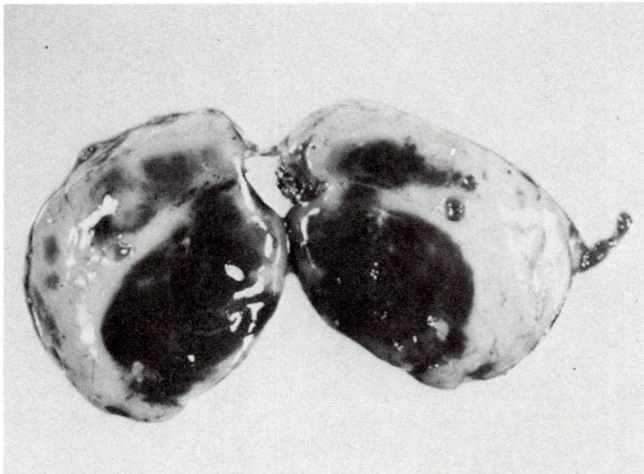

Fig 4–3.—In most cases, encounter and discovery of a parathyroid adenoma and three normal glands is curative.

thymic fat pad through the cervical approach, and often this technique is rewarding (Fig 4–4).

If four parathyroid glands are encountered and each appears to be either normal or only slightly enlarged, subtotal resection can take place following parathyroid biopsy examinations. If all four glands are biopsied, and the pathologist confirms that hyperplasia appears to be the diagnosis, a reexamination of the four biopsied glands is carried out, and those that appear the largest or nonviable following biopsy are selected for total excision. Approximately three and a half gland reduction is usually suggested for the primary management of parathyroid hyperplasia, but this can also be recommended in another way by reducing the total parathyroid mass to approximately 100 mg. One hundred milligrams is just over twice the size of the normal parathyroid gland, and, for safety, two glands may be excised, and 30- to 50-mg remnants of two others left in situ with marking clips attached. Some investigators advocate total parathyroidectomy and transplantation of parathyroid tissue to a more accessible spot than the neck so that serial parathyroid reduction can take place. More recently, cryopreservation of parathyroid tissue has been successful with in vitro testing of responsiveness to rule out autonomy. Transplantation of hyperfunctioning parathyroid tissue has occurred,[9] and some unfortunate patients are afflicted by an unnatural disease—recurrent hyperparathyroidism with hyperfunctioning parathyroid tissue in the neck and arm. The treatment for hypoparathyroidism may be a more satisfactory way to deal with this un-

TABLE 4–2.—PROCEDURE FOR SEARCH FOR FOURTH GLAND

I. Intraoperatively
   Pathologist's report confirms 3 glands
   Parathyroid "map" indicates position of missing gland
   Search posterior thyroid capsule in this position
   Examine "mirror image" position opposite confirmed gland
   A. If superior gland:
      Search above superior thyroid pole, taking down superior thyroid artery
      Palpate tracheoesophageal groove
      Explore retroesophageal area
      Dissect carotid sheath on suspected side
      Perform thyroidotomy
   B. If inferior gland:
      Trace any branches of inferior thyroid artery
      Palpate submanubrial space
      Tease up thymic fat pad
      Perform limited thyroidectomy in area where gland is missing
   C. Cyclic AMP urinary excretion monitoring
   D. If convinced that there is no evidence of additional parathyroid tissue in neck, *close!* *No* indication for sternotomy at a primary exploration.

II. Postoperatively
   A. Test for persistent hypercalcemia
   B. CAT and ultrasonic scanning
   C. Venous sampling and venography
   D. Arteriography
      1. If adenoma encountered in neck—cervical reexploration
      2. If mediastinal adenoma with inferior thyroid arterial blood supply—cervical reexploration
      3. If mediastinal adenoma with internal mammary arterial blood supply—embolize

usual problem than transplantation of autonomous parathyroid tissue. The in vitro studies that are being reported for confirmation of parathyroid suppressibility will be helpful in selecting patients for parathyroid transplantation.

POSTOPERATIVE CARE AND DRUG MANAGEMENT

If, after all of the techniques described in the intraoperative half of Table 4-2 have been exhausted, no adenoma is encountered, the surgeon may have reached the conviction that there is no evidence of additional parathyroid tissue in the neck. In such a case, closure is the next step. There is *no* indication for sternotomy at the time of primary exploration, since there are successful alternatives that may be employed for both diagnostic localization and therapy for ectopic adenomas outside the reach of the surgical field via the cervical incision. If the patient has persistent or early recurrent hypercalcemia that is convincing evidence of continued hyperparathyroidism, scanning and venous sampling tests may be carried out. If arteri-

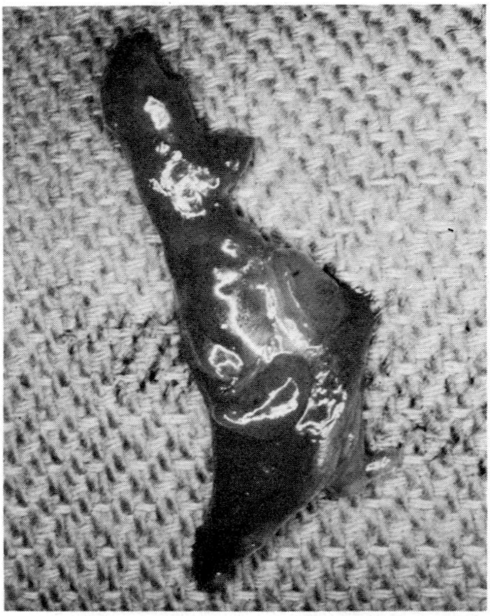

Fig 4–4.—If an ectopic parathyroid adenoma is found in the mediastinum suspended from its inferior thyroid artery blood supply, it can be mobilized into the neck through the cervical incision as seen in the instance of this intrathymic parathyroid adenoma.

ography is performed, ectopic, and particularly mediastinal, adenomas may "light up." If the mediastinal adenoma is superior and appears to be receiving its blood supply from the inferior thyroid artery, cervical reexploration can be carried out and the adenoma retrieved through this cervical approach (Fig 4–5).

If the mediastinal adenoma appears to have its arterial blood supply from the internal mammary artery, the diagnostic arterial catheter can be used for treatment of this ectopic adenoma using a technique that is an attractive alternative to sternotomy. Embolization by means of the arteriographic catheter has been a successful method of ablation of mediastinal parathyroid adenoma. This percutaneous technique may be accompanied by less morbidity than a sternum-splitting reoperation.[7]

FOLLOW-UP AND SPECIAL CONSIDERATIONS

Hyperparathyroidism is the common feature in both MEA-I and MEA-II. If there is a family history of confirmed diagnosis of either MEA-I or II, or if there is a family history of peptic ulcer disease, diarrhea, and other

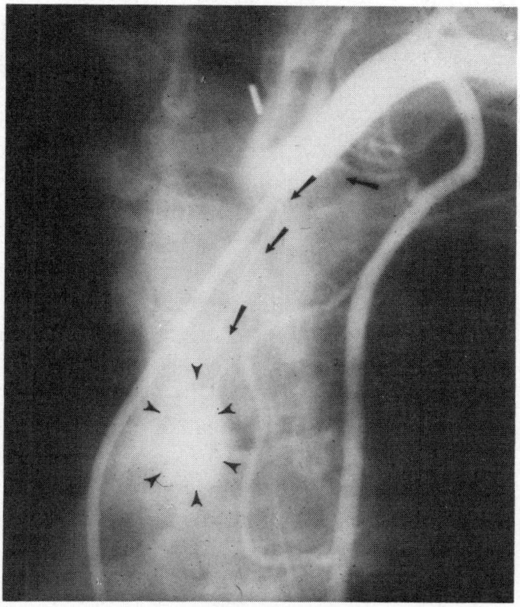

Fig 4–5.—Arteriographic appearance of an ectopic adenoma persistent after cervical exploration. Some mediastinal adenomas may be treated by embolization via the arteriographic catheter.

evidence of pancreatic islet cell tumor, skull films should be obtained, and serum gastrin and cortisol levels should be tested. No abnormality is expected primarily in the adrenal glands with MEA-I syndrome, but a pituitary adenoma that displaced the function of the anterior pituitary may lead to panhypopituitarism and an addisonian crisis during or after an operation for hyperparathyroidism. Even if the serum gastrin is elevated, it is important to carry out the parathyroid exploration to relieve the patient's hyperparathyroidism, since the serum gastrin may respond to the fall in serum calcium anticipated after successful parathyroidectomy. As remarked in the preceding chapter on the exploration of thyroid mass lesions, if hyperparathyroidism is part of the MEA-II syndrome, the cervical exploration is deferred until a pheochromocytoma can be ruled out. A careful examination of the thyroid is always possible during parathyroid exploration, and there may be encounter with thyroid pathology—follicular or other benign thyroid adenomas are found in many instances, and thyroid carcinoma in up to 7% of cases in whom no thyroid pathology is suspected. The common axiom is that if a patient has hyperparathyroidism with a palpable nodule in the neck, the nodule is most likely to be of thyroid rather than parathyroid origin. An incidental encounter with thyroid pathology during parathyroid exploration allows the treatment of both disorders, and thyroidectomy increases the exposure to the areas where parathyroid glands may be hidden.

One of the consequences of successful parathyroid excision that may be expected is hypoparathyroidism. Particularly after the excision of a large adenoma, the hypocalcemia may come on quickly and be profound. Patients are carefully monitored after parathyroid exploration, and at least twice daily serum calciums are drawn for the first 48- to 72-hour period. We do not treat "numbers in the blood" but treat symptomatic hypocalcemia. For tetany, the calcium is administered parenterally, and oral calcium supplementation is begun. In many instances, this may need to be supplemented with vitamin D if the patient remains symptomatic while receiving calcium feeding only. While monitoring the serum calcium, the vitamin D and calcium supplementation can be tapered, and the parathyroid remnants regain their effectiveness in sensing serum calcium and responding with appropriate parathyroid hormone synthesis and release.

A special group of patients of interest to the author is a small personal series of nonagenarians who proved to have hyperparathyroidism. It was the opinion of the referring physicians that this diagnosis was not a significant one in the multiple problems lists of these aged patients, each of whom was confined to a nursing home and suffered from cloudy mentation, incontinence, and inability to care for herself. A review of the records of all of these patients showed that they had long-standing hypercalcemia and biochemical patterns of primary hyperparathyroidism. After some effort, both family and physicians were convinced that there might be some benefit achieved from parathyroid exploration, which was described to them as an operation of minimal morbidity that could be tolerated by such persons of advanced age. Several of the patients achieved remarkable improvement postoperatively, including clearing of mentation in most of the patients, capability of self-care and a return to continence in all of them, and even discharge from nursing care facilities in one-third of these patients. It is stressed that hyperparathyroidism is a source of multiple functional problems, and that relief of hyperparathyroidism may make more manageable the other multiple problems uncovered in a review of systems that had been worsened by the compromised reserves in elderly individuals.

The operative treatment of hyperparathyroidism is very gratifying if the preoperative diagnosis is convincing and the cervical exploration is successful in identifying all parathyroid tissue. Particularly if an adenoma is removed, the patient may experience an immediate resolution of the hypercalcemia in a long-term cure. For those instances in which all the parathyroid tissue is not identified and confirmed histologically, and postoperative hypercalcemia is persistent, specialized techniques of localization and possibly additional methods of treatment of ectopic hyperfunctioning parathyroid tissue are called upon for adjunctive management of persistent hyperparathyroidism.

REFERENCES

1. Reeves C.D., Palmer E., Bacchus H., et al.: Differential diagnosis of hypercalcemia by the chloride/phosphate ratio. *Am. J. Surg.* 130:166, 1975.
2. Thalassinos N.C., Joplin C.F.: Failure of corticosteroid therapy to correct the hypercalcemia of malignant disease. *Lancet* 2:537, 1970.
3. Maselly M.J., Lawrence A.M., Brooks M., et al.: Hyperparathyroid crisis. *Surgery* 90:741–746, 1981.
4. Lemann J. Jr., Donatelli A.A.: Calcium intoxication due to primary hyperparathyroidism. *Ann. Intern. Med.* 60:447, 1964.
5. Clark O.H., Way L.W.: The hypercalcemic syndrome: Hyperparathyroidism, in Friessen S.R. (ed.): *Surgical Endocrinology*. Philadelphia, J.B. Lippincott, 1978, chap. 16.
6. Oyama T.: Parathyroid, in *Anesthetic Management of Endocrine Disease,* New York, Springer Verlag New York, 1973, chap. 7.
7. Geelhoed G.W., Doppman, J.L.: Embolization of ectopic parathyroid adenomas: A percutaneous treatment of hyperparathyroidism. *Am. Surg.* 44:71, 1978.
8. Schaefer C.J., Columbani P.M., Geelhoed G.W.: Absorbable ligating clips. *Surg. Gynecol. Obstet.* 154:513, 1982.
9. Brennan M.F., Brown E.M., Marx S.J., et al.: Recurrent hyperparathyroidism from an autotransplanted parathyroid adenoma. *N. Engl. J. Med.* 299:1057, 1978.

5 / The Carcinoid Syndromes

MANAGEMENT PROBLEMS

Problems for the patient with carcinoid syndrome include instability of the circulation, hyperreactivity of the bronchial air passages, heart failure from endocardial lesions, nutritional disorders from vitamin deficiency, disorders of intestinal and hepatic function, diarrhea, and the discomfort of flushing and other cutaneous manifestations of the carcinoid syndrome. A major patient problem, even absent from the carcinoid syndrome, is the metastatic spread of this oncologically malignant neoplasm.

The physician's problems in management include localization and removal or control of the primary tumor, the distinction of the different types of carcinoid syndromes and their mediators, appropriate surgical and drug therapy in endocrinologic control. The physician must also be aware of the association of carcinoid syndromes with other endocrinopathies and multiplicity of primary carcinoid tumors, as well as an association with other nonendocrine tumors. Management of the carcinoid syndromes includes oncologic considerations of the malignancy of the carcinoid tumor, as well as endocrinologic control of the systemic manifestations of carcinoid's endocrine mediators. However, the majority of carcinoid tumors do not produce significant endocrinologic disorders, particularly those that are not metastatic and a further subgroup that does not produce the carcinoid syndrome even when metastatic. Patients with the carcinoid syndrome call for an exercise of many of the management techniques described in this chapter, since the tumor is often slow-growing, and its chief morbidity may be products of its persistent endocrine function.

CARCINOID TUMORS, HORMONES, AND SYNDROMES

Carcinoid tumors have been described as "missing links between benign and malignant tumors."[1] Carcinoid tumors arise from the Kulchitsky's cells that are scattered through the linings of GI, respiratory, and genitourinary epithelium. These carcinoid cells share the APUD properties that enable them to synthesize and release a variety of amine and polypeptide endocrine products. Although the oncologic behavior of the carcinoid tumors may vary from the classic patterns of either benign or malignant tumors, their endocrine properties make possible distinctive physiologic abnormalities associated with these tumors that must be anticipated and managed.

When clinical patterns of endocrine manifestations called "carcinoid syndrome" form the presenting complaint, the carcinoid tumor is usually metastatic. For the amine components (serotonin and 5-hydroxytryptophan) to be active in the clinical patterns of vasomotor and skin changes that form part of the carcinoid syndrome, they must reach the systemic circulation. The liver and lungs degrade these amines through the action of the enzyme monoamine oxidase (MAO). For primary carcinoid tumors in the GI tract, endocrine secretions are picked up in the portal system and delivered to the liver (rich in MAO), where they are metabolized to the end-product of these amine hormones, 5-hydroxyindoleacetic acid (5HIAA). 5HIAA is released into the systemic circulation, but is not endocrinologically active,[2] being only excreted as a diagnostic marker of the carcinoid tumor's presence. If carcinoid metastases are present in the liver, the active form of the carcinoid endocrine secretions find their way into the systemic circulation, where they may exhibit their hormone effect. Venous blood would contain higher quantities of carcinoid hormones than arterial blood, because the lung also contains MAO and clears much of the amine hormones delivered to it. This fact may explain the anatomical distribution of one pathologic characteristic of carcinoid syndrome: endocardial lesions are often present, but usually predominantly on the right side of the heart. If the primary carcinoid tumor is in the tracheobronchial tree, then similar lesions may be found in left- and right-sided chambers of the heart.

Carcinoid hormones are produced by the totipotential APUD enzymes of the carcinoid cell. These hormones include serotonin, 5-hydroxytryptophan, kallikrein and kinins, histamine, prostaglandins, and a number of further peptide mediators.

Serotonin is the mediator often thought of as the definitive hormone of carcinoid syndrome. Many of the symptoms of carcinoid syndrome, however, are not well correlated with the serotonin levels, and cannot be reproduced by injection of serotonin.

5-Hydroxytryptophan is produced by carcinoid tumors that lack decarboxylase. This is the case with gastric carcinoid tumors, which have a different type of cutaneous flush than the gut carcinoids. The metabolic end-product of both serotonin and 5-hydroxytryptophan is the 5HIAA, which is used in diagnostic screening for carcinoid.

Kallikrein and kinins are a significant part of several carcinoid syndromes, and are the dominant features of bronchial carcinoids.

Histamine is released from some foregut carcinoids and may be the reason that peptic ulcer is associated with carcinoid syndrome in these instances.

Prostaglandins, ACTH, growth hormone, prolactin, and a dozen peptide mediators have been isolated from the carcinoid syndrome products and have been found in the carcinoid tumors and the bloodstreams of patients who bear these carcinoid tumors.

Carcinoid tumors in some locations, such as the appendix, rarely spread, and some malignant carcinoid tumors from other locations, such as the rectum, even if widely metastatic, do not result in carcinoid syndrome.

Carcinoid syndrome is actually a collection of clinical syndromes. Each syndrome reflects the predominant variety of the hormones secreted by the polypotential carcinoid cell. Carcinoid tumors originating in different organ sites may give rise to differing carcinoid syndromes, which will make management different, largely due to the differing dominance of several species of carcinoid humoral agents.

The management problem in carcinoid syndrome will be focused on the most frequent and most severe of the patient complaints. A chief complaint in the carcinoid syndrome is vasomotor instability. The carcinoid patients will also have discomfort from flushing attacks, diarrhea, wheezing, abdominal and musculoskeletal pain, and vitamin deficiency. Specific types of carcinoid syndromes will have specialized problems outlined below, some of which are amenable to specific treatment.

DIAGNOSIS

The measurement of the serotonin metabolite, 5HIAA, is the single best diagnostic indicator of carcinoid syndrome that may be used for screening purposes. Serum tests may include direct assay of the serotonin, histamines, prostaglandins, or kinins that circulate in the active carcinoid syndrome. To stimulate release of these hormones, provocative tests have been devised using alcohol or calcium.[3]

An important provocative test is the epinephrine test, which is also instructive in the problems of managing the carcinoid patient intraoperatively. In the carcinoid patient, a positive test to epinephrine injection is the induction of flushing and a fall in blood pressure. This paradoxical hypotension in response to epinephrine may be a result of the release of kinins into the circulation. To either administered or endogenous epinephrine, this "bradykinin shock" will be a major response to be anticipated in the carcinoid patient undergoing an operation or stress.

Localization of the primary tumor is less important in cases that present with carcinoid syndrome, since the tumor will be metastatic, and often the metastases are much larger than the primary tumor itself. Furthermore,

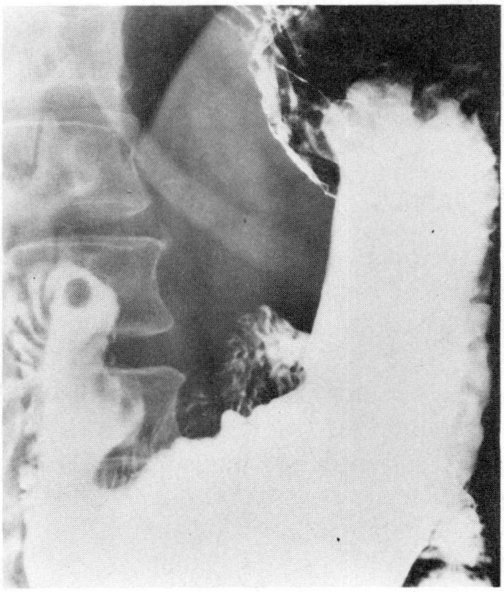

Fig 5–1.—Upper GI contrast series reveals a primary duodenal carcinoid (confirmed by endoscopic resection) in a patient with carcinoid syndrome.

unlike other endocrine tumors, localization is less a problem in the carcinoid tumor since operative exploration will be the best method of locating the tumor, and it is often multiple or associated with other tumors, making preoperative localization studies less important. Contrast series may show the origin of the tumor in the gut (Fig 5–1) or endoscopy and chest x-ray may be useful in the preoperative work-up.

PREOPERATIVE PREPARATION

Cardiography and cardiologic consultation are important in the preoperative evaluation of the patient with carcinoid syndrome to look for evidence of endocarditis, particularly in manifestations of tricuspid or pulmonic valvular stenosis. Phonocardiography, echocardiography, or scanning may be helpful in assessment following clinical indicators of right-sided heart failure.

Diarrhea is a major debilitating problem for the carcinoid patient. Crampy abdominal pain goes along with changes in transit time and fluxes across the wall of the intestine. Careful replacement of the fluid and electrolyte loss of this secretory diarrhea is important preoperatively. Since the diarrhea and borborygmi seem to be correlated with serotonemia, serotonin antagonists may be helpful in controlling these symptoms preoperatively.

Carcinoid syndrome patients may have a pellagra-like vitamin deficiency. Tryptophan is being diverted from niacin and protein synthesis to the production of the amine hormones of the carcinoid syndrome. At least 50 mg of niacin should be supplemented in the daily intake of the carcinoid patient.

Hypoalbuminemia and right-sided heart failure may lead to edema in the carcinoid patient, and IV albumin may be required preoperatively to substitute for deficient protein synthesis.

ANESTHESIA MANAGEMENT

A working knowledge of carcinoid pharmacology is essential for the intraoperative management of the carcinoid patient. Two major hazards the carcinoid patient faces in the operating room are bronchoconstriction and hypotension.

BRONCHOSPASM.—Bronchoconstriction is anticipated from the release of several of the amine and peptide hormones in the carcinoid syndrome. Endotracheal intubation and monitoring of ventilatory pressures can signal this endocrine effect on airway smooth muscle. But, to overcome bronchoconstriction, commonly used bronchodilators are *contraindicated*. All of the β-adrenergic agonists or drugs that cause endogenous catecholamine release will lead to the second major complication, hypotension (see "bradykinin shock" below).

Somatostatin has been shown to improve symptoms caused by some GI peptide hormones by inhibiting their action or release.[4] It has been reported that IV injection of 250 μg of somatostatin can relieve the bronchoconstriction of carcinoid syndrome for up to 90 minutes after injection.[5] The use of this counteracting hormone may be a useful adjunct in the airway management of the carcinoid patient.

BRADYKININ SHOCK.—The paradoxical response to β-adrenergic agonists in giving rise to hypotension was the positive end point in the provocative epinephrine test for carcinoid. This same paradoxical response may occur with administration or release of endogenous catecholamines during the stress of the operation. Drugs or anesthetics that mimic β-adrenergic activity or stimulate it (Table 5–1) are strictly contraindicated in carcinoid patients, since they cause release of kinins. The effect of bradykinin release

TABLE 5–1.—MAJOR PERIOPERATIVE PROBLEMS

	CONTRAINDICATED	INDICATED
Bronchoconstriction	Bronchodilators	Somatostatin
Bradykinin shock	Catecholamines or Catecholamine releasers	Crystalloid and colloid volume

may be to slow or to stop the heart. This bradykinin shock is a serious consequence of operations in carcinoid patients.

Hypotension may normally occur in patients during operation; however, possibly because of the volume deficit of diarrhea that has not been adequately repleted or because of vasodilatation this intraoperative hypotension is doubly serious in the carcinoid patient. In addition to the perfusion deficits of hypotension, reflex release of catecholamines is triggered and the further compounding of bradykinin shock is added. Rapid volume replacement should be employed (with consideration of the patient's possibly impaired cardiac status), often using albumin or other colloid for expansion. If a vasoconstrictor is necessary, an α-agonist, such as phenylephrine, may be used with care.

Curare may give rise to bronchoconstriction of its own action and should be avoided, but pancuronium[6] appears to be a satisfactory relaxant in carcinoid patients. The analgesic agent that appears to be best tolerated by carcinoid patients is fentanyl.[7]

In the postanesthetic period, the CNS may be depressed, with slow arousal, as a direct pharmacologic effect of serotonin circulation.

OPERATIVE TECHNIQUE

Patients with carcinoid syndrome generally benefit from operative resection of carcinoid tumor, even if the operation is designed for subtotal tumor reduction. Nearly all operations on patients with carcinoid syndrome should be considered palliative, with reductive surgery as an adjunct to drug therapy. Carcinoid tumor is one of the rare instances in which limited excision of metastatic disease in the liver may be beneficial. Resection of the primary tumor site and the regional nodes that may be involved (Fig 5–2) not only further reduces tumor burden, but also may treat or prevent intestinal obstruction that may occur from the "desmoplastic" response to carcinoid tumors that penetrate the serosa.

Of particular importance during laparotomy is a careful exploration in search for multiple primary sites of carcinoid tumor, present in up to 25% of patients with small-bowel carcinoids.[2] Moreover, up to 55% of patients may have a second, nonendocrine, cancer that must be sought during the operation, which is the best examination of the GI tract possible at that time in the patient's disease. An adjunctive technique in the control of metastatic carcinoid syndrome that may be helpful in some patients is hepatic artery ligation to relieve symptoms and control the rate of growth of the metastasis.

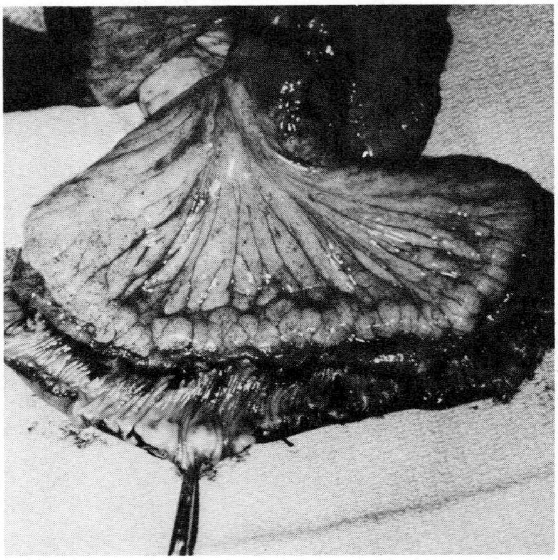

Fig 5–2.—Resection of a segment of ileum with multiple carcinoid tumors and large lymphatic metastases in a patient who presented with carcinoid syndrome.

POSTOPERATIVE CARE AND DRUG MANAGEMENT

Pharmacology directed at carcinoid symptoms may target the serotonin pathway, the kinins, agents that reduce host response, or antimetabolite chemotherapy (Table 5–2).

Diarrhea is largely a serotonin-dependent symptom, and drug management employs antiserotonin agents. Methysergide is a widely used serotonin antagonist, and cyproheptadine is both antiserotonin and antihista-

TABLE 5–2.—DRUG MANAGEMENT

PROBLEM	DRUG
Nutrition	Niacin
Diarrhea	Antiserotonin agents
	Methysergide
	Cyproheptadine
	Empiric drugs
	Opiates, codeine
Flushing	Phenoxybenzamine
	Glucocorticoids
(Gastric carcinoid	flush—methyldopa)
Peptic ulcer	Cimetidine
	Antihistamines

mine. Experimental drugs are being developed that inhibit synthesis of serotonin by affecting tryptophan hydroxylase or that act as "false messenger" tryptophan analogs.

Flushing is largely a kinin-dependent symptom, and drug management inhibits kinin release or dampens kinin effects. Phenoxybenzamine is useful as a blocking agent. Glucocorticoids may reduce flushing frequency and severity. Newer evidence shows that flushing from some forms of carcinoid syndrome may be inhibited by H_1 and H_2 receptor antagonists, implicating histamine as the principal mediator of this form of flushing.[8]

Prostaglandin inhibitors do not seem to relieve flushing, but somatostatin may inhibit the carcinoid flush as well as bronchoconstriction.[4, 9] Methyldopa is used for the flushing in gastric carcinoid syndrome, since methyldopa is a decarboxylase inhibitor, and tumors that secrete 5-hydroxytryptophan are successfully inhibited by the use of this drug.

Phenothiazines and antihistamines have been used empirically as well as direct GI motility inhibitors, such as opiates or codeine, for diarrhea. Drug therapy for cytotoxicity is mainly the function of streptozocin, useful in many of the APUD-cell malignancies.

FOLLOW-UP AND SPECIAL CONSIDERATIONS

Patients' conditions can be monitored by symptoms and by 5HIAA excretion.

Carcinoid syndrome is often a concomitant of another nonendocrine tumor, and a careful surveillance should be maintained to find and treat the second cancer as early as possible. Carcinoids also tend to be multiple, and the patient should be checked at intervals to find out if any new primary carcinoids have developed in the same system, such as in the GI tract.

Carcinoid tumors may exist as part of an MEA-I syndrome, and may also be associated with several other endocrinologic abnormalities that should be looked for during follow-up, including hyperparathyroidism, evidence of Cushing's syndrome, pancreatic islet cell neoplasms, or peptic ulcer.

REFERENCES

1. Geelhoed G.W.: Carcinoid: The cell, tumor and syndromes, in Pilch Y., das Gupta T. (eds.): *Surgical Oncology*. New York, McGraw-Hill Book Co., 1981, chap. 32.
2. Kaplan E.L.: The carcinoid syndromes, in Friesen S.R. (ed.): *Surgical Endocrinology*. Philadelphia, J.B. Lippincott Co., 1978, chap. 11.
3. Kaplan E.L., Jaffe B.M., Peskin G.W.: A new provocative test for the diagnosis of the carcinoid syndrome. *Am. J. Surg*. 123:173, 1972.
4. Frolich J.C., Bloomgarden Z.T., Oates J.A., et al.: The carcinoid flush: Provo-

cation by peritogastrium and inhibition by somatostatin. *N. Engl. J. Med.* 299:1055, 1978.
5. Klapdor R.: Effects of somatostatin on bronchial constriction in a patient with carcinoid syndrome. *N. Engl. J. Med.* 302:464, 1980.
6. Dery R.: Theoretical and clinical considerations in anaesthesia for secreting carcinoid tumors. *Can. Anaesth. Soc. J.* 18:235, 1971.
7. Mason R.A., Steane P.A.: Carcinoid syndrome: Its relevance to the anesthetist. *Anesthesia* 31:228, 1976.
8. Roberts L.J. II, Marney S.R., Oates J.A.: Blockade of the flush associated with metastatic gastric carcinoid by combined histamine H_1 and H_2 receptor antagonists. *N. Engl. J. Med.* 300:236, 1979.
9. Bloomgarden Z.T., Rabinowitz D., Oates J.A.: Carcinoid flush: Role of gastrin and somatostatin. *N. Engl. J. Med.* 300:624, 1979.

6 / Insulinoma

MANAGEMENT PROBLEMS

The patient with hyperinsulinism develops hypoglycemia, and the immediate effect of hypoglycemia is reflected in two nervous systems: CNS hypoglycemia leads to irritability, disorientation, behavioral disturbance, diplopia, changes in vision, drowsiness and seizures, and finally coma; autonomic nervous system symptoms include tachycardia, diaphoresis, apprehension, and nausea. The loss of mental function and coordination is the chief embarrassment to the patient, who may be thought to be intoxicated; moreover, as hypoglycemia progresses and recurrent episodes occur, this "insulin shock" can cause irreversible CNS deficits.

The problem for the physician in management of insulinoma is, first, recognition of the signs of hypoglycemia and its confirmation in the fasting state in adults. When fasting hypoglycemia is confirmed, among the differential diagnoses that may lead to this condition, endogenous hyperinsulinism must be proved to be concurrent with the hypoglycemia. With confirmation of the diagnosis, the problem becomes one of localization of the tumor and its surgical removal with medical management of some forms of persistent hyperinsulinism.

THE INSULINOMA—HORMONES AND SYNDROME

Insulinoma is the most common of the functioning islet cell neoplasms, and among the most gratifying to detect and treat. It is by no means rare and is almost always a curable or manageable problem that would be otherwise life-threatening.

The average normal adult human pancreas weighs about 70 gm, almost all of which is exocrine parenchyma, with the exception of from 1 to 2 million clusters of endocrine cells that Langerhans called "islets." These islets collectively weigh approximately 1 gm, and an average islet weighs approximately 1 μg. Several cell types have been identified histologically in human islets and have been arbitrarily labeled according to their staining characteristics. When the islet cells were identified as endocrine organs that secreted peptide mediators, the products of these "insula" became "insulin." It was subsequently found that the β islet cell produced the hypoglycemic hormone that retained the name insulin, which was the major hormone regulating carbohydrate metabolism.

The β islet cells synthesize a large polypeptide molecule, proinsulin, which then undergoes proteolytic division into active insulin and a connecting peptide (C-peptide). Both C-peptide and the double-chain polypeptide insulin are secreted from β cell granules and should rise together during pancreatic islet stimulation, as occurs during hyperglycemia. Occasionally, the β islet cells escape control of this glucose feedback inhibition, either because of neoplastic transformation (insulinoma) or diffuse hyperplasia. Measurement of proinsulin in the bloodstream has been helpful in studying patients with insulinoma, since they uniformly have been found to have high circulating serum proinsulin.[1] It has also been suggested that patients with malignant insulinomas may have a higher percentage of proinsulin values than patients with benign insulinomas.

Measurement of the β islet cell polypeptides has facilitated the diagnosis of insulinoma. The C-peptide fragment can be used also as a marker of overproduction of the products of β islet cell synthesis, as well as the direct assay of insulin and proinsulin. Since the C-peptide is a marker of β islet cell output, but without endocrine function, it may be helpful in ruling out other causes of hypoglycemia. Furthermore, because of its inert marker function, it can be measured in patients who are diabetic and who require insulin administration that would cross-react with insulin assays run by radioimmunoassay. In normal individuals, exogenous insulin infusion should cause a suppression of the β islet cell secretion, as should hypoglycemia; but in persons with insulinoma, continued secretion monitored by C-peptide levels would be strong supporting evidence of an autonomous insulinoma.

The syndrome that results from hyperinsulinism is a reflection of an excess of *two* hormones: a surge of insulin release gives a direct hypoglycemic effect, particularly on the CNS, but it is also a potent stimulus to epinephrine release. One patient in the author's experience was referred for evaluation of a possible pheochromocytoma, since she had paroxysms of tachycardia, diaphoresis, and behavioral disturbance, following which her measured urinary catecholamines were elevated. During diagnostic testing for a pheochromocytoma (see chap. 10), she was found to have normal serum catecholamines, but fasting reproduced the "attacks."

The clinical evidence of this hypoglycemic syndrome was popularized by Whipple in the description of a clinical triad.[2] "Whipple's triad" clinically described patients with insulinoma who had (1) hypoglycemic attacks after fasting or exertion, (2) fasting blood sugar levels of less than 50 mg/dl, and (3) relief of symptoms with administration of carbohydrates.

Whipple's triad remains the classic clinical criterion by which patients are screened to select those who will undergo the current definitive tests for hyperinsulinism—fasting blood samples for simultaneous measurement of glucose and an inappropriately elevated insulin immunoassay (glucose-insulin ratio).

DIAGNOSIS AND DIFFERENTIATION FROM OTHER FORMS OF FASTING HYPOGLYCEMIA

Hypoglycemia in the adult may be on the basis of postabsorptive reactions, such as the "dumping syndrome" postgastrectomy; deficient glucose production, as in the alcoholic patient who has cirrhosis of the liver and cannot mobilize glycogen for a glucose reserve; overutilization of glucose in the fasting state (which would include the insulinoma); and pharmacologic or toxic agents that depress blood sugar. If one distinguishes only *fasting* hypoglycemia in the adult, hyperinsulinism would lead the list that includes other causes such as nonendocrine tumors, Addison's disease, liver disease, such as cirrhosis, and late starvation when energy reserves may be exhausted.[3]

Patients with insulinoma typically present with interesting personal vignettes: a very distinguished gentleman became quite combative and hostile when dinner was late; a young man became "giddy" following jogging in lieu of lunch; a middle-aged woman was very embarrassed because her co-workers stated she always "acted like a child" in the late morning before lunch break; a young woman was distressed because she was gaining weight as a result of multiple caches of sweet snacks that she had stashed around the house and office, which she would consume to prevent "lightheadedness."

On the basis of such histories and the strong evidence of Whipple's triad in each of these patients, they were admitted for the definitive diagnostic test for hyperinsulinism as inpatients. The definitive test is quite simple and involves fasting, sometimes for a prolonged period. Blood samples are taken at intervals and whenever the patient complains of hypoglycemic symptoms. The blood samples are assayed for blood glucose and insulin levels to determine the ratio of glucose to immunoreactive insulin and proinsulin during the fast. An inappropriately high insulin level during hypoglycemia is diagnostic if the possibility of exogenous insulin injection has been eliminated. There are provocative tests other than fasting to prove elevated insulin and low blood sugar levels, but all these studies are *inpa-*

tient studies, since dangerous hypoglycemia may result. Tolbutamide, glucagon, or L-leucine can be given as a stimulus to insulin release, but this test must be done under a physician's supervision for the hospitalized patient, and aborted immediately if the patient becomes stuporous. Through the same needle that drew the blood samples during the positive provocative tests, a 50% glucose solution is given by IV push to stop the test.

Suppression tests include IV injection of diazoxide, which should depress insulin release in the hypoglycemic patient. Failure to do so implies an autonomous source of insulin secretion. Some patients, particularly medical personnel, might try to produce factitious hypoglycemia by self-injection of insulin, but this can be checked by assaying the bloodstream for C-peptides, which should not be present in commercial insulin preparations and should be released from an insulinoma. Insulin antibodies also build up in response to exogenous insulin, and these may be assayed as well.

In the patient with Whipple's triad who has an inappropriate elevation of serum insulin during fasting hypoglycemia, the next step is tumor localization. This is a meticulous process, since most insulinomas are typically quite small. High-resolution techniques are needed for the detection of pancreatic islet cell tumors that may be producing severe symptoms from a lesion 0.5 cm in diameter. The single best study for insulinoma localization is a selective pancreatic arteriogram, usually augmented by subtraction

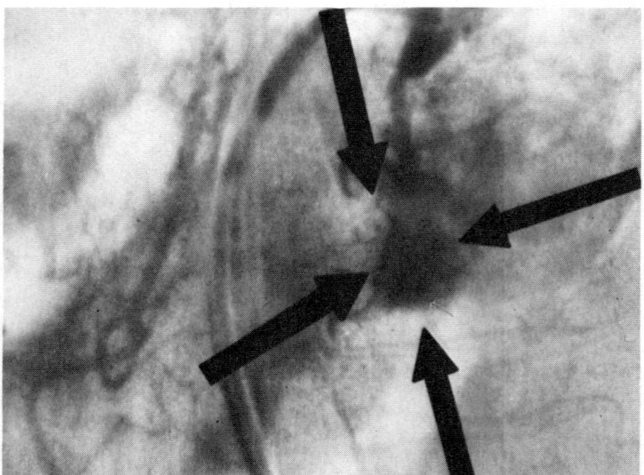

Fig 6–1.—Selective pancreatic arteriogram with subtraction technique is the highest resolution method of insulinoma localization preoperatively. Insulinomas are better visualized by this localization technique than any other islet cell tumors.

views. Pancreatic islets are quite vascular, and an islet cell tumor of the insulinoma type may show up as a tumor blush; single, ectopic, and multiple lesions may be demonstrated with the arteriographic technique. In two patients in the author's experience, an initial arteriogram was negative, and other noninvasive studies, such as CAT scan and sonogram, were not helpful either. But as symptoms persisted and the patient was admitted for operation, a repeated selective angiogram preoperatively was able to demonstrate the lesion. Insulinomas are the best visualized of the islet cell pancreatic tumors, and the best resolution of these tumors is accounted for by angiography (Fig 6–1). A new technique may be helpful for some individuals who fail to demonstrate insulinoma on arteriography despite convincing clinical evidence of hyperinsulinism. This technique involves the percutaneous and transhepatic cannulation of the portal vein[4] and selective sampling along the course of the splenic vein (Fig 6–2). A site of very high insulin concentration if the sampling technique is constant suggests a focal insulin source within the drainage field mapped by this portal catheter. This technique was misleading once in the author's experience when the

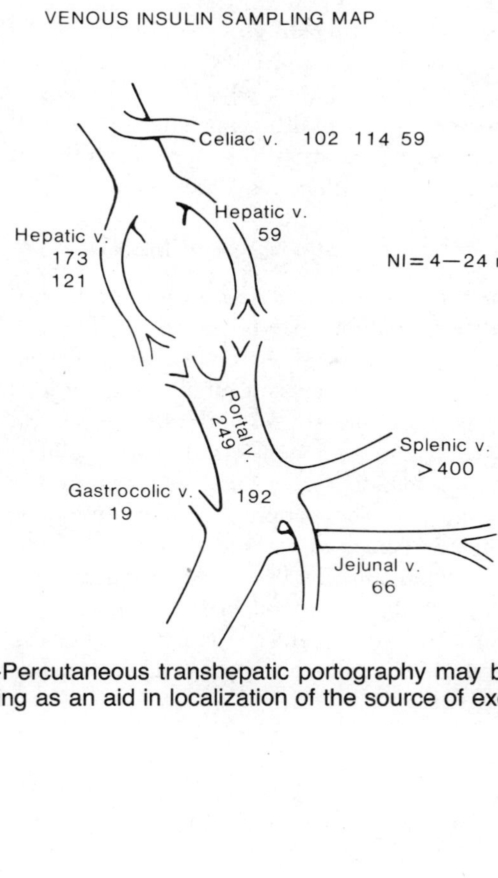

Fig 6–2.—Percutaneous transhepatic portography may be used for selective insulin sampling as an aid in localization of the source of excess insulin release.

rate of blood drawing and other sampling techniques were not constant. The advent of digital subtraction angiography may prove to be useful in vascular tumor localization within the pancreas, but has been used only once in the author's experience because of its recent installation in our institution.

PREOPERATIVE PREPARATION

A typical order for anyone about to undergo laparotomy would routinely be written "NPO after midnight." This brings the patient to the operating room in the fasting state, which (as already noted) is a potent provocative test for insulinoma. Furthermore, the patient then undergoes anesthesia, which obliterates the CNS signs of dangerous hypoglycemia. It is standard practice to employ between-meal snacks and continuous absorption of carbohydrate and protein, which can be converted to carbohydrate slowly by gluconeogenesis. The importance of this continuous nutrition is based in the lack of any energy stores in the CNS. The brain has no glycogen, and depends on continuous bloodstream delivery of glucose and oxygen for adequate aerobic metabolism. Interruption of either of these substrates for energy may mean the rate-limiting step in survival. It is for this reason that when the patient with insulinoma stops oral intake, IV glucose is administered continuously. For some patients who may not have a focal insulinoma, but some degree of suppressibility as in microadenomatosis, diazoxide is a valuable preoperative preparation to suppress insulin release. Corticosteroids may be given for their gluconeogenic activity.

ANESTHESIA MANAGEMENT

Premedication for the insulinoma patient should be limited to the use of atropine.[5] The insulinoma patient may be drowsy and is usually quite sensitive to barbiturates and narcotics. A corticosteroid preparation may be administered in much the same way as it might be given for the addisonian patient undergoing an operative stress, and using the same doses. Ether and cyclopropane have hyperglycemic effects, and are useful inhalation gases. Hypoglycemia in the unconscious patient can be recognized sometimes from its epinephrine stimulation. The patient with sweating, pallor, and ECG changes may be in insulin shock under anesthesia.

Monitoring of the blood glucose is possible in the operating room by using glucose oxidase test tapes dipped in the patient's serum to be sure that an adequate concentration of glucose is getting into the bloodstream. Newer glucose-monitoring insulin pumps are also available as "servosystems" for glucose regulation.

The glucose infusion that was started when the patient was made NPO is continued on a constant delivery rate throughout the operation (Fig 6–3). This not only assures the operative team that the patient may be getting an adequate glucose level for protection of the CNS, but also aids in an indirect bit of evidence to confirm that the insulinoma has been resected. As seen in Figure 6–3, the blood sugar level rose after the pancreatic islet cell tumor was removed. Some surgeons suggest that a servomechanism can be set up in the operating room resembling an artificial β cell which could monitor blood glucose, vary the rate of glucose infusion, and even shift to insulin injection when the blood sugar rises. The author has not yet seen the need for this automated technology, and the only confidence in a continuous delivery rate of IV glucose and frequent blood glucose monitoring is to insure that the patient's nervous system is not being starved of the only substrate it can use. Although it may seem definite to see a reassuring pattern of hyperglycemia occur after tumor resection, this may be misleading. Manipulation and dissection around the tumor may stimulate a surge of insulin into the bloodstream that can occur more quickly than reflected by the glucose monitoring methods. So, the intraoperative blood glucose curve is a supporting document of evidence that may rule out profound hypoglycemia, particularly if the patient does not have a rapid arousal following the operation, but cannot be the sole crutch upon which the determination of tumor extirpation rests.

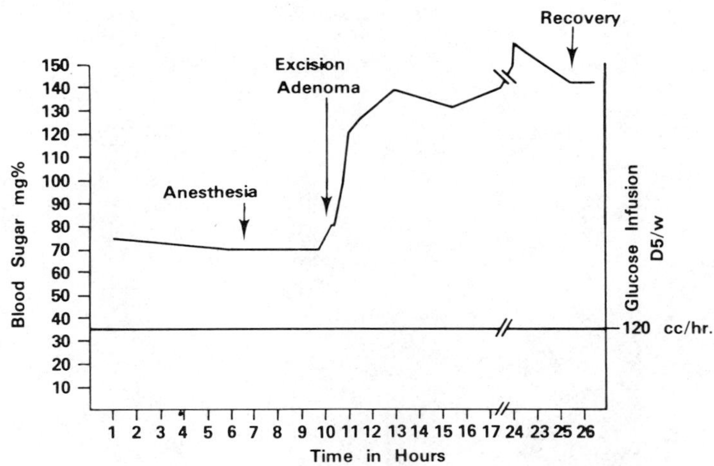

Fig 6–3.—Constant intravenous glucose infusion during anesthesia maintains safe blood glucose levels, which rise when the insulinoma is resected.

OPERATIVE TECHNIQUE

Operation is the ultimate "localization procedure" in diagnosis, and usually the definitive step to end the treatment of insulinoma. The lesser sac is entered and the retroperitoneum exposed with careful palpation of the entire anterior surface of the pancreas. A Kocher's maneuver is performed to lift the duodenum and get bidigital palpation of the head of the pancreas. The inferior border of the pancreas is lifted for palpation along its length. Special attention is paid to any area of hypervascularity shown on the preoperative angiogram.

Typically, pancreatic palpation for discovery of an insulinoma is like *The Princess and the Pea*. In the normal pancreas the firm nubbin of islet tissue is remarkable. If there has been any degree of previous exocrine pancreatic inflammation and fibrosis, the "ropey" consistency of the pancreas makes the palpation technique more difficult. If a small tumor is found, enucleation is often possible with gentle dissection of the exocrine parenchyma away from the islet cell tumor and application of ligating clips to minimize the rupture of pancreatic ductules and somewhat lessen the risk of pancreatic fistula formation (Fig 6–4). If the solitary adenoma is found, the entire extent of the pancreas must still be carefully searched, because insulinoma may occasionally be multiple or may occur in ectopic locations outside the pancreas.

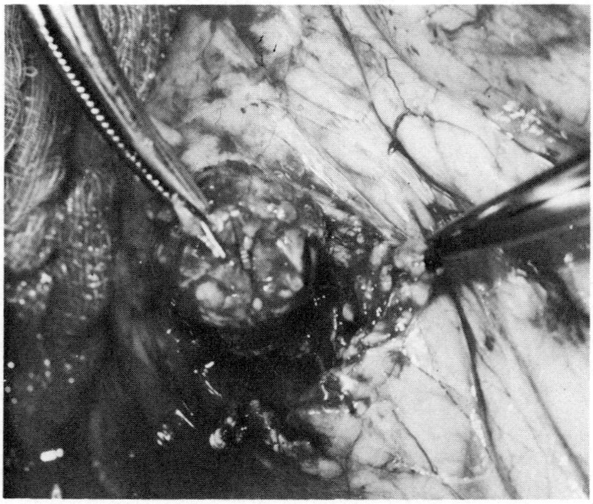

Fig 6–4.—The majority of insulinomas are small, solitary, and benign, and resection may only involve enucleation of the adenoma from the surrounding pancreatic parenchyma.

The pathologist's consultation is very important in insulinoma exploration, and a discussion of the facts of the case with the pathologist preoperatively will help in the histologic confirmation by frozen section intraoperatively. If no adenoma can be palpated, sequential "blind" pancreatic resection may become necessary. Since insulinomas are rather even in their distribution frequency in the pancreas, the "blind" resection of the pancreas begins with the easier forms of pancreatic resection. Usually this means distal pancreatectomy sequentially toward the portal and mesenteric vessels, until the pathologist announces a positive finding on frozen section examination. If the pancreas that was carefully palpated within a duodenal sweep by Kocher's maneuver and the usual sites of pancreatic ectopia have been examined, and subtotal pancreatectomy has been carried out, one of three possible reports may be issued on frozen section examination. Either a small adenoma has been found, microadenomatosis or nesidioblastosis[6] has been found, or no abnormal islet tissue has been encountered. At that point, a check on the intraoperative blood glucose curve may also reveal no change, but the glucose monitoring system is not a flawless indicator of success. It is recommended that the operation be terminated at this point, since permanent section pathology examination may reveal a very small adenoma that could be overlooked on frozen section. The author knows of one instance in which a pancreatic exploration was negative for abnormality through the final pathology report and was followed by a curative long-term response by the patient.

Total pancreatectomy, or pancreaticoduodenectomy, is probably never indicated at the initial exploration, since other alternatives are available for the management of persistent symptoms. Postoperative hypoglycemia can be medically managed, and an adenoma that was initially overlooked may grow to visibility on a later repetition of the angiogram.[7]

Problems of this nature are rare, since the great majority of insulinomas are very rewarding for surgical treatment. Unlike other islet tumors (see chaps. 7 to 9), the majority of insulinomas are small, solitary, benign, and both visible on arteriography and curable on limited pancreatic resection.

POSTOPERATIVE CARE AND DRUG MANAGEMENT

The patient postinsulinoma resection may have hyperglycemia, rarely indicating treatment with insulin, since hyperglycemia is the appropriate stimulus to the β islet cells in the remaining pancreas. If glycosuria and ketoacidosis ensue, very light doses of insulin may be given to the patient. The most useful drug in following up patients who have symptoms of persistent or recurrent hypoglycemia is diazoxide. This drug can be "titrated" to the patient's needs, although it does nothing to the growth of the benign or malignant residual insulinoma. Cytotoxic chemotherapy employing streptozocin has met with some success in reducing islet cell growth and thereby dampening the hypoglycemic effect.[8, 9]

In the majority of the patients following insulinoma resection, the glucose tolerance test curve gradually returns toward normal. When metastatic malignant insulinoma is encountered, debulking metastatic disease surgically at a "second-look" operation reduces symptoms and prolongs life.

FOLLOW-UP AND SPECIAL CONSIDERATIONS

Any patient with insulinoma should have a skull film or pituitary tomogram done to check for any evidence of MEA-I. The most serious consequence of a pituitary tumor that may not be recognized preoperatively is its displacement of normal ACTH secretion; a preoperative check on cortisol can exclude this possibility, or routine use of perioperative stress-dose steroids in insulinoma resections may avoid any addisonian crisis from panhypopituitarism, although principally given for its gluconeogenic effect. In later follow-up of the insulinoma patient, particularly the patient who has a positive family history, a check on other pancreatic islet cell syndromes should include serum gastrin and human pancreatic polypeptide studies, since other islet cell tumors might arise later in the patient or in the patient's family.

Insulinoma is an eminently treatable disease, well worth searching for, confirming, and correcting, since patients with the insulinoma syndrome are not only embarrassed by their CNS dysfunction, but are at grave risk to life should fasting be prolonged and the hypoglycemia make the patient unable to feed or to account for himself. The successful correction of endogenous hyperinsulinism protects the patient, prevents irreversible brain damage, and returns the patient to physiologic control of carbohydrate metabolism.

REFERENCES

1. Kaplan E.L., Lee C.-H.: Recent advances in the diagnosis and treatment of insulinomas, Symposium on Endocrine Surgery. *Surg. Clin. North Am.* 59:119, 1979.
2. Whipple A.O., Frantz V.K.: Adenoma of islet cells with hyperinsulinism. *Ann. Surg.* 101:1299, 1935.
3. Fajans S.S., Floyd J.C. Jr.: Fasting hypoglycemia in adults. *N. Engl. J. Med.* 294:766, 1976.
4. Ingemansen S., Kuhl C., Larsson L., et al.: Localization of insulinomas and islet cell hyperplasia by pancreatic vein catheterization and insulin assay. *Surg. Gyn. Obstet.* 146:725, 1978.

5. Oyama T.: Anesthetic management of insulinomas, in *Anesthetic Management of Endocrine Disease*. New York, Springer-Verlag New York, 1973.
6. Harness J.K., Geelhoed G.W., Thompson N.W., et al.: Nesidioblastosis in adults: A surgical dilemma. *Arch. Surg.* 116:575, 1981.
7. Harrison T.S., Child C.G. III, Fry W.J., et al.: Current surgical management of functioning islet cell tumors of the pancreas. *Ann. Surg.* 4:485, 1973.
8. Schein P.S., DeLellis R.A., Kahn C.R., et al.: Islet cell tumors: Current concepts and management. *Ann. Intern. Med.* 79:239, 1973.
9. Moertel C.G., Hanley J.A., Johnson L.A.: Streptozocin alone compared with streptozocin plus fluorouracil in the treatment of advanced islet cell carcinoma. *N. Engl. J. Med.* 303:1189, 1980.

7 / Zollinger-Ellison Syndrome

MANAGEMENT PROBLEMS

The patient's problems in Zollinger-Ellison syndrome include symptoms of recurrent or persistent peptic ulcer disease and diarrhea. Coupled with these symptoms, which are the chief causes of morbidity, is the malignant potential for this pancreatic islet cell tumor. Although the tumor may be slow-growing, it can cause a patient's death from metastatic disease.

The management problem for the physician is how to control the functional problems that arise from the excess of gastrin secretion, and how to control the underlying islet cell tumor itself. The management objectives of the Zollinger-Ellison syndrome have changed rapidly over the recent past, with the advent of new management methods and the reports of the experience of several groups with quite different treatment goals.

THE SYNDROME: THE GASTRINOMA, GASTRIN, AND THE ULCEROGENIC SYNDROME

The original report of Zollinger and Ellison in 1955[1] described patients with the following ulcerogenic islet cell tumor triad (compared with the original Whipple's triad for insulinoma): (1) fulminating ulcer diathesis, (2) gastric hypersecretion, and (3) non-β islet cell tumor. A later clinical feature was added to this triad, with a description of secretory diarrhea as part of the Zollinger-Ellison syndrome.

Later reports, however, have shown that gastrinoma may be present without the extreme intractibility of the ulcer disease, and in fact, some patients with proven gastrinoma have only diarrhea with no proof whatsoever of ulcer disease.[2]

A comparison may be drawn with pheochromocytoma for screening purposes: peptic ulcer disease is a prevalent problem in the developed world, and it has been subsequently learned that Zollinger-Ellison syndrome patients may present with a wide variety of subtle symptoms including some that run in families. But the gastrinoma is far less common than peptic ulcer disease, probably representing less than 0.5% of the causes of peptic ulcer. In chapter 10, it is pointed out that hypertension is a prevalent disease, and that pheochromocytoma has a wide variety of features in its clinical presentation; however, not more than 0.1% of patients with hypertension have it on the basis of this etiology. It is more important to discover the pheochromocytoma, however, since it constitutes a life-limiting threat which is potentially curable in the great majority of cases treated. It may be less important to discover gastrinoma as early as possible, for, since methods of management over a prolonged period are available, the disease is less frequently regarded now as the atypical fulminant peptic ulcer disease that was the immediately life-limiting threat, and the potential for cure of the gastrinoma itself is limited.

Although a gastric hormone in the control of acid production had been postulated for 50 years, it was not until five years after the clinical description of the Zollinger-Ellison syndrome that gastrin was identified, and only within the last decade has a radioimmunoassay for gastrin become widely available for clinical testing. Rather than screening all patients with any degree of peptic ulcer syndromes with serum gastrin determinations, gastrinoma should be suspected in a more limited group of patients. These include patients with unusual ulcer disease: very young ulcer patients, those with chronic ulcer symptoms, patients with severe complications of ulcer disease, and those patients with very high gastric acid determinations. Another group of patients in whom it is beneficial to determine serum gastrin

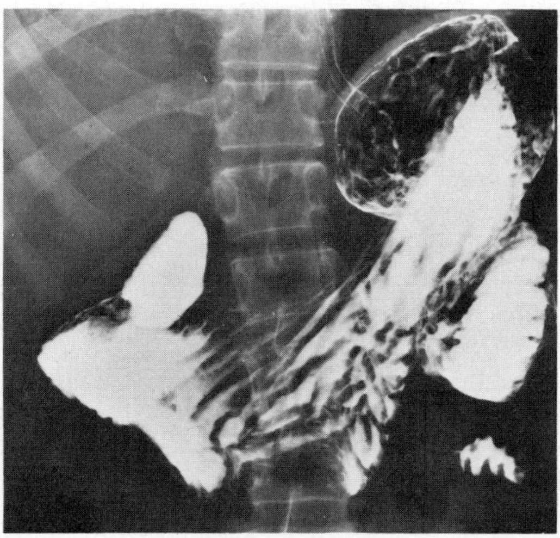

Fig 7–1.—Appearance of gastric hyperrugosity on barium study strongly suggests an increased parietal cell mass. Jejunal ulceration is a pathognomonic radiographic feature of Zollinger-Ellison syndrome.

levels and to suspect the Zollinger-Ellison syndrome are those patients with unusual x-ray film changes, including gastric hyperrugosity (Fig 7–1), duodenal nodularity and severely deformed duodenal bulb, and intestinal hypermotility. A nearly pathognomonic sign of Zollinger-Ellison syndrome on upper GI series is ulceration of the jejunum just distal to the ligament of Treitz.

Patients who should have the potential of Zollinger-Ellison syndrome considered are also those who have unexplained diarrhea, other endocrinopathy, or a strong family history suggestive of MEA-I (see chap. 14).

Another unusual feature of the Zollinger-Ellison syndrome that has more recently been understood is the slow progression of the disease over the course of many years. Spontaneous remission may develop, and one clinical syndrome may yield to another in the APUD-cell abnormalities that may be sequential, particularly in the families with MEA-I that may have Zollinger-Ellison syndrome as part of the hereditary endocrinopathy.

DIAGNOSIS: CONFIRMATION OF HYPERGASTRINEMIA AND GASTRINOMA LOCALIZATION

For islet cell tumors of the insulinoma variety, there was noted an urgency in confirming the diagnosis because of the danger of hypoglycemia and a strong incentive for precision localization, since the majority of insulinomas are solitary, benign, and curable by local excision. By contrast, the biologic nature of gastrinoma is quite different. The majority are *malignant, multifocal,* and *metastatic* when first encountered at operation. Since the option for curative treatment is limited, the gastrinoma is slowly progressive, and the usual manifestations of the syndrome are not life-threatening, there is less urgency to the diagnosis of gastrinoma than insulinoma.

In screening patients with unusual ulcer disease, the diagnosis of peptic ulceration is usually made with radiographic contrast study for those with chronic ulcer symptoms. Gastric dilatation and prominent rugal folds in the unobstructed stomach suggest a greatly increased parietal cell mass (see Fig 7–1). Duodenal distortion and a "cobblestone" appearance from mucosal edema and hypertrophy of Brunner's glands may support the suggestion of Zollinger-Ellison syndrome, particularly if there is megaduodenum and evidence of hypermotility. In addition to these radiographic signs, the historical information is helpful in selecting those patients whose peculiar ulcer history, with or without diarrhea as an additional feature, should suggest gastrinoma. However, not all patients with peptic ulcer disease and high gastrin determinations qualify for the Zollinger-Ellison diagnosis. This combination can also be seen with retained excluded antrum, carcinoma of the stomach, and renal failure. Gastrinase is a renal enzyme, and interpretation of serum gastrin must be made cautiously in the patient with impaired renal function. This deficit in gastrinase activity may be significant in the ulcer disease that is more frequent in patients with renal failure. Even if primary hypergastrinemia is proven, it may not be originating in the focal gastrinoma, but an entity known as antral G-cell hyperplasia also may give rise to excess gastrin.

To distinguish hypergastrinemia from other causes, further diagnostic testing is required. Overnight gastric acid output and basal and maximal stimulated acid output can suggest gastrinoma if the basal:maximal ratio is greater than 0.6. Stimulation tests have been devised to provoke increased gastrin release that can be measured and, indirectly, an increase in acid production. Calcium or secretin infusions cause a marked increase in gastrin release in gastrinoma patients, whereas the same tests in peptic ulcer patients show gastrin unchanged to decreased. The challenge of a protein test meal can be carried out, which markedly increases the serum gastrin in peptic ulcer patients, but shows no change in the patients with Zollinger-Ellison syndrome. The secretin stimulation test would be chosen in the author's institution as preferable to the other stimulation tests.

Localization of gastrinoma is very unrewarding, since the tumor is rarely a focal solitary neoplasm. The localization study that is discouraging is the same arteriography that proved to be most successful in localization of insulinomas. Sonography or CAT scanning can detect multiple masses, particularly metastatic lesions adjacent to the pancreas or in the liver. The single localization study that might be carried out for the benefit of identification of a small subgroup of Zollinger-Ellison syndrome patients is duodenal endoscopy. This localization test is important not because of the high yield of submucosal duodenal gastrinomas, but because this group of patients may constitute the rare exception to the rule of gastrinoma multiplicity. Duodenal endoscopy might discover the few patients with solitary gastrinomas in the duodenal wall that are resectable for cure.

PREOPERATIVE PREPARATION

Preoperative preparation depends to some extent on the nature of the operation intended. Nearly all patients with Zollinger-Ellison syndrome will now be prepared with cimetidine for a prolonged period of time either as a method of gastric acid output inhibition in anticipation of operation or as a substitute for it. Standard antacids and anticholinergics are employed to reduce the pain of ulcer and the crampy discomfort of the diarrhea associated with gastrinoma. A very important feature in the preoperative preparation is the passage of a nasogastric tube which is placed to suction. Besides decreasing the gastric acid volume delivered to the gut, this simple maneuver makes an important distinction between the diarrhea of Zollinger-Ellison syndrome and other diarrheogenic syndromes based on pancreatic islet cell tumors (see chap. 8). Prolonged gastric suction, however, may lead to hypochloremic metabolic alkalosis from the high volume gastric acid output that is lost.

ANESTHESIA MANAGEMENT

A preoperative check on the patient's acid-base and electrolyte status might allow preanesthetic correction of hypochloremic metabolic alkalosis. For those patients with gastrinoma suspected of being familial, skull x-rays and a cortisol determination will rule out the potential for addisonian crisis in patients undergoing a major gastric or pancreatic operation with panhypopituitarism. A careful check on the serum calcium level is very important, since an elevated calcium determination might suggest hyperparathyroidism, which should be corrected first by an operation with much lower morbidity and mortality than a major resection of the stomach or pancreas. A correction of hypercalcemia may lead to suppression of endogenous hypergastrinemia and a reduction of the peptic ulcer symptoms or diarrhea in Zollinger-Ellison syndrome, particularly in patients with MEA-I.

OPERATIVE TECHNIQUE

A major controversy in the management of the Zollinger-Ellison syndrome now involves the role of surgery in the control of the primary gastrinoma and its functional consequences. Rational therapy for a hyperfunctioning endocrine adenoma would be extirpative surgery. To remove the very few gastrinomas that are not metastatic, Whipple pancreaticoduodenectomy would be the primary extirpative treatment—a major operation that is doomed to failure in most cases of Zollinger-Ellison syndrome and is overtreatment of the few that it would help.

"Target treatment" seems somewhat irrational, but as it originally evolved, it was less incapacitating to the patient to attack the target organ rather than the primary source of the pathophysiology, either ablating the target organs or interfering in their hyperfunction. Originally the high mortality from Zollinger-Ellison syndrome was related to the sequelae of gastric acid hypersecretion in untreated or inadequately controlled cases more than to the presence of metastatic malignant disease. The management of Zollinger-Ellison syndrome that evolved was consequently directed to the control of the "benign," but lethal, complications of gastric hypersecretion rather than a "cancer operation" on the pancreas or its metastases. Since circulating gastrin has little effect in the absence of the stomach, total gastrectomy eliminated the end-organ through which the gastrinoma expressed most of its morbidity and mortality. Originally, mortality statistics for Zollinger-Ellison syndrome were very high unless total gastrectomy had been performed in all patients.

A turnabout in the management methods occurred with the advent of successful drug therapy to control gastric hypersecretion. Since gastric acid secretion is mediated—both by increased gastrin and vagal stimulation—through histamine release, blockade of the receptors for histamine activation in the stomach has been successful in the control of gastric acid hypersecretion. Blockade of the H_1 receptors with classic antihistamines was limited in its effectiveness, but H_2 receptor blockade has been shown to be very effective. Earlier H_2 receptor antagonists had shown toxicity, particularly with agranulocytosis; cimetidine was developed with little marrow suppression to limit its use, although it has other toxicity which is less severe but not negligible.

With H_2 receptor antagonists available for the control of gastric hypersecretion, the stomach no longer has to be ablated to insure a lower postoperative mortality and morbidity from recurrent gastrinoma acid-mediated complications. Surgical exploration could revert back to a primary focus on the site of the gastrinoma, establishing the gastrinoma diagnosis histologically, resection of tumor at the few favorable sites where the gastrinoma may be solitary and resectable, such as the wall of the duodenum or the tail of the pancreas, the staging of metastatic disease, and reduction of tumor burden when possible for palliation that can be done safely. Gastrectomy is no longer the primary operative treatment of choice for Zollinger-Ellison syndrome. A 25-year review of the clinical experience with gastrinoma has been published by the original observer,[3] which suggests that lesser gastric acid-reduction operations may have some role adjunctively with the availability of receptor blockade.

New indications for gastrectomy are based in the variability of cimetidine control, the differential assay of gastrin species that suggest the biologic behavior of the tumor, and the age of the patient. Total gastrectomy cannot be abandoned in the primary treatment of gastrinoma, but the indications for its performance have been more narrowly defined.[3] Attention is also being refocused on the role of limited pancreatic resection for reduction of gastrinoma burden in those instances in which the stomach may remain in situ during drug control of the functioning residual tumor. Proximal gastric vagotomy may reduce the need for cimetidine to control gastric acid output, and makes the patient more sensitive to lower doses of this drug following selective vagotomy.[4]

POSTOPERATIVE CARE AND DRUG MANAGEMENT

Patients who have had total gastrectomy for control of Zollinger-Ellison syndrome are capable of gaining weight and returning to electrolyte, acid-base, and nutritional balance postoperatively. It is said that patients undergoing total gastrectomy for Zollinger-Ellison syndrome tolerate the operation with better nutritional rehabilitation than those who have had total gastrectomy for cancer,[5] although, in the limited experience of the author, this has been true only for those whose gastric carcinomas have proved to be uncontrolled.

Serum gastrin determinations can be made as a marker to follow the progress of the pancreatic tumor, and elevation of gastrin over 1,000 pg/ml is indication for repeated CAT scanning and arteriography. Cimetidine treatment is not required in the absence of the stomach. Antitumor chemotherapy may take the form of streptozocin and fluorouracil.

Gastrinoma is a persistent problem that should be thought of more in terms of management and control than cure. One of the original patients in the first description of the syndrome continues to have elevated gastrin determinations 25 years postoperatively, although she continues to do well. Two patients in the author's experience who have had only diarrhea as a major manifestation of gastrinoma have failed localization studies, have declined operation, and are being followed up receiving cimetidine therapy alone. Over a prolonged period, the drug dosage has been modified, and anticholinergic agents added to adjust control periodically, but for the time this management appears to be adequate for control of their symptoms if not for the underlying tumor. Management methods for Zollinger-Ellison syndrome are still in evolution, and drug therapy in lieu of operation must still be tentatively called the new standard of care for this disorder. If patients evolve the indications suggested earlier as more closely defined indications for operation, the options remain open as to the selection of operation on the target organ or the primary tumor with anticipation of long-term drug control of the functional consequences of circulating gastrin.

FOLLOW-UP AND SPECIAL CONSIDERATIONS

The gastrinoma patient is followed up for life. Dr. Zollinger has used the adage, "Once a tumor, always a tumor."[6] Not only must they be followed up for evidence of increased activity or frank metastatic spread of the disease, but they must also be screened for the development of additional endocrinopathies, especially other islet cell neoplasms and MEA-I features in the patient and the family.

REFERENCES

1. Zollinger R.M., Ellison E.H.: Primary peptic ulcerations of the jejunum associated with islet cell tumors of the pancreas. *Ann. Surg.* 142:709, 1955.
2. Fang M., Ginsberg A.L., Glassman L., et al.: Zollinger-Ellison syndrome with diarrhea as the predominant clinical feature. *Gastroenterology* 76:378, 1979.
3. Zollinger R.M., Ellison C.E., Fabin P.J., et al.: Primary peptic ulcerations of the jejunum associated with islet cell tumors: Twenty-five-year reappraisal. *Ann. Surg.* 192:422, 1980.
4. Richardson C.T., Feldman M., McClelland R.N., et al.: Effect of vagotomy in Zollinger-Ellison syndrome. *Gastroenterology* 79:682, 1979.
5. Deveney C.W., Deveney K.S., Way L.W.: The Zollinger-Ellison syndrome—23 years later. *Ann. Surg.* 178:188, 1978.
6. Zollinger R.M.: The ulcerogenic (Zollinger-Ellison) syndrome, in Friesen S.R. (ed.): *Surgical Endocrinology*. Philadelphia, J.B. Lippincott Co., 1978, chap. 14.

8 / The Diarrheogenic Syndromes

MANAGEMENT PROBLEMS

The patient with this islet cell tumor has a very inconvenient, metabolically dangerous, and potentially lethal dysfunction in this secretory diarrhea. Secondary symptoms from fluid and electrolyte loss include muscular cramps and weakness.

The problem in management for the physician is to control the continuing loss in fluid and electrolytes while carefully replenishing the depleted body stores of these essential nutrients. The physician must also differentiate secretory diarrhea from malabsorption and a wide variety of etiologies and mediators among the former in order to design specific surgical and drug management. The acuity of the management problem is underscored by the fact that 10% of the patients with "pancreatic cholera" died during the phase of preoperative management following diagnosis.[1]

THE TUMOR, HORMONES, AND SYNDROMES OF PANCREATIC CHOLERA

The diarrheogenic syndromes are perhaps the best example of the totipotential endocrine capabilities of APUDomas. From this pancreatic islet cell tumor can issue multiple mediators in different predominance, making possible different specific therapy in selected instances. Furthermore, in natural progression or under the pressures of therapy, the APUD-cells may modify their secretion patterns and produce somewhat different clinical effects.

The diarrheogenic syndrome has been known to be associated with a non-β islet cell tumor since shortly after the description of the Zollinger-Ellison syndrome, and was first thought to be a variant of it. It became known as the Verner-Morrison syndrome following their description of the hypokalemia and achlorhydria prominent as part of the syndrome, although later it was determined that hypochlorhydria is a more nearly correct characterization of these patients. Most of the patients that have been described are middle-aged women, and the common features of the diarrhea have given rise to an acronym "WDHA" for watery diarrhea, hypokalemia, and achlorhydria. The watery diarrhea is nearly invariably the presenting feature before any pancreatic abnormality is known; it may begin intermittently and become nearly continuous as the pancreatic tumor progresses. The clinical effect is a very high volume of up to 10 L/day in its most malignant form, justifying the term "pancreatic cholera." The volume of this diarrhea is remarkable, but so is its electrolyte content, with approximately 300 mEq of daily potassium loss and a high quantity of bicarbonate. The syndrome does not seem to be associated with crampy pain, since hypermotility is not a feature of the syndrome, nor is malabsorption or steatorrhea.

With the identification of the secretory nature of this diarrhea, a logical sequence would be to identify the cell of origin (like the β cell of insulinoma) and the hormone responsible for the clinical effect (like the insulin secreted by insulinoma). These attempts to isolate the hormone made by a specific cell have been frustrated, since multiple mediators exist within the diarrheogenic syndrome, the cell of origin remains obscure, and other APUDomas confuse the picture by causing clinically similar secretory diarrhea.

DIAGNOSIS

The differential diagnosis of diarrhea includes the broad categories of malabsorption of the fluids within the GI tract, increased intestinal motility and decreased transit time, and the endocrine diarrheas that are based in secretory hyperactivity. Endocrine diarrhea may be present in several distinct syndromes, including Zollinger-Ellison syndrome, carcinoid syndrome, medullary thyroid carcinoma, and some of the rare GI APUDomas that may be included with the WDHA syndrome.

Studies of fecal fat excretion, D-xylose absorption, and small-bowel biopsies may be normal in these patients, whereas serum studies reflect the effect of their body losses, showing hypokalemia, acidosis, prerenal azotemia from dehydration, and hypomagnesemia. Assays of circulating hormones may yield one, many, or no identifiable mediators in the patients with the active disease. Evidence for and against several hormones can be summarized [1] by listing gastrin, glucagon, and serotonin as unlikely mediators, equivocal evidence for secretin, and potential evidence for the vasoactive intestinal peptide (VIP),[2,3] human pancreatic polypeptide (HPP), and some species of prostaglandin.[4] No single hormone fulfills "Koch's Postulates" as an adequate etiologic agent to describe all of the features seen in each of the diarrheogenic syndrome patients.

An important differential diagnosis is made between the diarrhea seen in Zollinger-Ellison syndrome (see chap. 7) and the WDHA syndrome. As

TABLE 8–1.—ZOLLINGER-ELLISON VS. WDHA SYNDROMES*

FEATURE	ZES	WDHA
Diarrhea	Acid	Alkaline
Gastric volume	Increase	Normal
Gastric acid	Increase	Decrease
Nasogastric suction	Relief of diarrhea	No relief of diarrhea
Motility	Increase	Normal

*WDHA, watery diarrhea, hypokalemia, and achlorhydria syndrome. The simplest, most effective means of differentiating between the two syndromes makes use of nasogastric intubation.

shown in Table 8–1, the diarrhea is acid in Zollinger-Ellison syndrome, and the pH is alkaline for WDHA. The volume of secretion appears to be coming from the stomach for Zollinger-Ellison syndrome, and appears to be originating below the ligament of Treitz for WDHA. The single most important simple test to differentiate the two is the passage of a nasogastric tube. Aspiration of the contents of the stomach stops the diarrhea of Zollinger-Ellison syndrome, but has no effect on WDHA diarrhea.

PREOPERATIVE PREPARATION IN THE DIARRHEOGENIC SYNDROME

Nearly all of the attention in management of WDHA should be focused in preparation of the patient, with gradual and adequate repletion of the fluid and electrolyte loss as the first objective. These patients have suffered severe and prolonged dehydration with electrolyte depletion compounding a contracted fluid volume. The problems of the preoperative period have a higher mortality than does the operation, and correction of the fluid, electrolyte, and pH imbalance must take place with a special concern for the potassium deficit.

There is no method to accomplish swift potassium repletion safely, and these patients have had large daily deficits accumulating for extended periods. A deliberate and gradual potassium repletion is intended to equilibrate intra- and extracellular potassium by cautiously infusing potassium that must be delivered through the extracellular space. But potassium chloride should not be the electrolyte supplement chosen for this purpose, since the patients have lost very little chloride because of their relative hypochlorhydria. Hyperchloremic acidosis is the rule, and this may be made worse by potassium chloride infusion. If magnesium is not given simultaneously, tetany may result.

The safest way to provide necessary replenishment is in a metabolic unit, where patients' measured losses can be determined and a surplus of the potassium over this measured loss replaced while monitoring other changes in fluid and mineral metabolism.

ANESTHESIA MANAGEMENT

The principal concern of the anesthesiologic team is also the loss of salt and water, with its consequences for organ function. Besides the primary dehydration, acidosis, and azotemia, two target organs affected are the heart and kidneys. Hypokalemic myocardial dysfunction may be monitored on ECG, and nephropathy can result from the volume contraction and acidosis. Muscle weakness is a prominent feature of hypokalemic patients, and this problem has implications for the ability of these patients to manage the work of breathing and the ability to mobilize reserves in the stress of exertion. The more prolonged and thorough the preoperative preparation, the safer will be the anesthetic course.

OPERATIVE TECHNIQUE

WDHA tumors are typically larger than insulinomas, and localization has been less of a problem for this reason. Operative exploration for the tumor is much more gratifying than similar pancreatic exploration for gastrinoma. The majority of patients operated upon have benign adenomas which can be resected for cure, usually by subtotal pancreatectomy. This has involved distal pancreatic resection, removing the tail of the pancreas to the medial margin of the mesenteric vessels in two cases the author has seen, and in one instance, enucleation of a smaller mass from the head of the pancreas was adequate treatment to relieve symptoms.

POSTOPERATIVE CARE AND DRUG MANAGEMENT

It is interesting that the preoperative features of WDHA include the notable absence of gastric acid, whereas following curative resection, patients not only produce acid, but also may develop peptic ulceration. Antacids and H_2-receptor antagonists may be employed to minimize this postoperative complication. If the tumor is subtotally resected or metastases are present, several specific forms of drug therapy may be helpful in postoperative management. One patient with a metastatic tumor was seen to have relief of symptoms after intra-arterial streptozocin injected through a hepatic artery catheter left at the conclusion of an operation to reduce tumor. An interesting form of specific symptomatic relief can be given to those patients whose pancreatic cholera is based in a prostaglandin-predominant mediator, since prostaglandin-inhibiting drugs are available and have proven useful for control of symptoms.[4] Nonspecific therapy includes some palliation that is obtainable with corticosteroid treatment.

FOLLOW-UP AND SPECIAL CONSIDERATIONS

The WDHA may be part of generalized APUD neoplasm syndromes, such as MEA-I. In addition, the secretion from the tumor may be variable depending on as yet incompletely understood provocative stimuli, and specific agents may be developed to block the stimulants or inhibit their effect at the receptor site. A very aggressive expansion of clinical and biochemical APUD polypeptide research offers optimism for further understanding and control of this group of clinical syndromes.

REFERENCES

1. Jaffe B.M.: The diarrheogenic syndrome, in Friesen S.R. (ed.): *Surgical Endocrinology*. Philadelphia, J.B. Lippincott, 1978, chap. 15.
2. Ebeid A.M., Murray P.D., Fischer J.E.: Vasoactive intestinal peptide and the watery diarrhea syndrome. *Ann. Surg*. 187:411, 1978.
3. Bloom S.R., Gardner J.D.: The VIP controversy. *Am. J. Dig. Dis*. 23:370, 1978.
4. Jaffe B.M., Condon S.: Prostaglandins E and F in endocrine diarrheogenic syndromes. *Ann. Surg*. 184:516, 1976.

9 / Glucagonoma, Somatostatinoma, and Ectopic Hormone Sources

MANAGEMENT PROBLEMS

Patients with glucagonoma have weight loss, depression, mild diabetes, and a very unusual skin rash. The other patients with tumors discussed in this chapter generally have an undifferentiated tumor that may be metastatic and that causes functional endocrine problems as an incidental problem besides their oncologic major problem.

The management problem for physicians is the identification of those patient problems that signal an underlying disease that may be treatable and the recognition that some of these "paraendocrine" features may require symptomatic treatment for patient comfort in the face of an uncontrolled primary malignancy.

INTRODUCTION

For purposes of reference, the author has only seen one patient with glucagonoma, one with somatostatinoma, one other patient with a primary pancreatic islet cell tumor elaborating as yet unknown polypeptides, and two patients with pancreatic islet cell nesidioblastosis that elaborated multiple identifiable polypeptides. These anecdotal experiences are not presumed to be a base for generalization, with the exception of the striking features of some of the patients (such as the glucagonoma and its associated rash) that may aid others in the recognition of such a syndrome. However, patients are frequently referred for evaluation of paraendocrine syndromes that may resemble APUD-cell neoplasms that are reasonably well characterized. Each of these patients seems to be one-of-a-kind, but collectively they form additional evidence in support of the unifying APUD concept, and allow inference as to their management.

DIAGNOSIS

The glucagonoma syndrome appears in late middle age, in more women than men, and may show up as a pattern of mild diabetes, usually detected by an abnormal glucose tolerance curve rather than the complications of uncontrolled diabetes. The diabetes does not appear to be complicated by ketoacidosis, retinopathy, nephropathy, neuropathy, or small-artery disease, and the patients who present may have the diabetes discovered incidental to the remarkable skin rash, or the more general complaints of depression and weight loss. Occasionally, small doses of insulin may be necessary for the control of the diabetes, but most of the patients have elevations in their circulating insulin, as well as glucagon, which offsets the extremes of glucose intolerance.

The feature by which most of the cases have come to diagnosis and the nearly pathognomonic characteristic of glucagonoma is a skin rash. The rash appears over the perineum, lower abdomen, feet, and perioral areas with glossitis. Migration of this rash occurs in a pattern of spreading erythema, with healing following in the areas from which the rash has migrated.

Necrolytic migratory erythema (NME) is the name of this specific skin rash in glucagonoma. Its highly specific histologic appearance is seen if a skin biopsy is taken at the advancing edge of the lesions, showing necrolysis and pale staining of the upper epidermis and keratin separation in bullae. Often the active edges of the rash may be superinfected with fungus and bacteria, and some of the characteristic histologic appearance may lose distinctiveness. The majority of these patients have had severe depression, often seeming worse when the skin rash is most prominent, and regressing dramatically when the pancreatic tumor is resected. Many of the patients described have had deep venous thrombosis and several pulmonary emboli have occurred.

The classic presentation of glucagonoma is based on the NME rash, but without the rash, patient presentation may be indistinguishable from ordinary diabetes until the pancreatic tumor—usually malignant—appears, causing cachexia and depression. Sometimes, glucagonoma may appear in MEA kindreds, often due to islet cell hyperplasia or carcinoma, as well as adenoma, and these patients often lack the characteristic NME rash. The diagnostic test for glucagonoma is the skin biopsy with the confirmed NME and an assay for circulating glucagon, which is disproportionately high for the corresponding levels of insulin and glucose.

Somatostatinoma has only been known for a few years, and only a few patients have been described. From these anecdotal instances, however, there appears to be a general pattern of adult onset diabetes and gallstones. Most of the individuals had the D cell pancreatic islet tumor discovered at laparotomy for cholecystectomy. Somatostatinoma has been called the "inhibitory syndrome"[1] because of the somatostatin activity as an "endogenous cyanide." The inhibitory response of somatostatinoma seems to be selective, suppressing insulin and glucagon when excessive somatostatin is circulating from the tumors in the pancreas from which it has been isolated. Preoperative diagnosis is not likely in the majority of instances of somatostatinoma in the future, since the combination of diabetes and cholelithiasis is very common, and somatostatinoma is extremely rare. However, somatostatin plays an interesting hormonal role in the inhibition of other islet cell secretions, and may help us understand the modulation of secretion in other islet cell syndromes. As discussed in Chapter 5, some of the circulatory and bronchospastic features of the carcinoid syndrome might be controlled by the administration of somatostatin, and it may be that under normal physiologic circumstances, somatostatin may effect a "paracrine effect" that is seen in exaggerated form when the somatostatinoma is present.

Malignant tumors that arise from cells outside the APUD-cell line may occasionally give rise to one or more APUD-like hormones. One of the more common syndromes that results from this "tumor derepression"[2] is the "syndrome of inappropriate ADH" (SIADH). In this case, ADH is secreted by epithelial tumors in the airway or GI tract, kidney, or brain that is virtually indistinguishable from pituitary ADH. The "inappropriateness" of the ADH secretion leads to excessive water retention and symptoms of water intoxication, with serum sodium and osmolality markedly depressed. In the author's experience, the most frequently seen examples of SIADH occur in patients with bronchogenic carcinoma and metastatic epidermoid cancers of the head and neck. The diagnosis has usually been made by the serum sodium determination during water restriction, proving the inappropriate dilution of the plasma, rather than the more difficult assay for ADH.

Probably next in order of frequency of unusual "ectopic" hormone production is the secondary Cushing's syndrome that comes not from the secretion of steroids by unusual tumors, but by the synthesis of ACTH-like proteins which stimulate the adrenal cortex. Hyperpigmentation is often frequent in this ectopic hormone syndrome because of the similarity in function of melanocyte-stimulating hormone (MSH) and ACTH.

Nearly all of the polypeptide hormones described to this point and their consequent syndromes have been seen from ectopic production. In some very unusual neoplasms, usually of foregut origin, multiple hormones may be released and the consequent syndromes may overlap in their clinical presentations. Usually such neoplasms do not present management problems because of their endocrine features, as much as they cause concern about the malignant behavior of the primary tumor. However, the patient may have relief from the endocrine functions of these tumors through some of the same management methods as are outlined for the syndromes caused by nonectopic hormone hypersecretion.

PREOPERATIVE PREPARATION

For glucagonoma, somatostatinoma, and other rare primary GI polypeptide syndromes, the techniques of tumor localization and preparation for operation have been borrowed from the lessons learned from the more common pancreatic and other GI syndromes. These include localization by noninvasive scanning and arteriography. Diphenylhydantoin has been used for inhibition of some of the secretions from glucagonoma particularly, but the dangers of severe imbalance in glucose or mineral metabolism seen in such syndromes as that encountered with insulinoma or WDHA syndrome are not present for this group of neoplasms. Fluid and electrolyte balance are much more important with the SIADH, and fluid restriction and careful balance studies are done to control these patients, who usually do not come to operation for control of their syndrome as much as for potential extirpation of their primary malignant disease.

ANESTHESIA MANAGEMENT

No specific recommendations for the anesthetic management of glucagonoma or somatostatinoma may be generalized from the anecdotal experience; however, for those patients with some of the ectopic hormone syndromes, the endocrine hyperfunction may be the limiting step in operability for the primary tumor. For example, the patient who has a tumor secreting ADH or an ACTH-like substance will require correction of the abnormalities that stem from this hormone function before enduring the manipulation of the operation directed at the primary tumor.

OPERATIVE TECHNIQUE

Operation directed at the control of the primary pancreatic tumors (glucagonoma and somatostatinoma) is not often curative, but frequently is beneficial. Subtotal pancreatectomy or "debulking" in cases of either tumor have given the patients improved quality of and prolonged life. Particularly in the case of glucagonoma, palliative operation has been accompanied by a fall in glucagon levels and a dramatic—nearly instantaneous—improvement in the NME skin rash. Even with the loss of a considerable quantity of the pancreas, glucose tolerance may be improved.

In the syndromes of inappropriate or ectopic hormone production, operation is often directed at the primary tumor—frequently in lung or the GI tract—and such operations are rarely curative, but may be followed by immediate relief of the endocrine syndromes with an increase in patient comfort.

POSTOPERATIVE CARE AND DRUG MANAGEMENT

Patients who have had subtotal resection of their disease have occasionally benefited from antimetabolite chemotherapy, particularly with streptozocin. However, particularly in the glucagonoma syndrome, it must be remembered that this form of drug therapy also effects β islet cells of the pancreas, and after treatment both insulin and glucagon may decrease, and glucose tolerance may be affected adversely. Zinc supplementation has been suggested for the NME rash. The single instance in the author's observation of subtotal resection of glucagonoma resulted in a notable improvement, nearly within 24 hours of the operation, and, within days, resolution of both the rash and depression.

FOLLOW-UP AND SPECIAL CONSIDERATIONS

A general judgment cannot be imposed on the scattered anecdotal instances of some of these unusual pancreatic or ectopic hormone syndromes. However, a great deal of information may be extracted from the instances of cases observed and small series of those reported to help in understanding polypeptide hormone properties whether originating appropriately or inappropriately. As in the other cases discussed in previous chapters, the MEA syndromes (see chap. 14) may involve one of these more unusual pancreatic or GI-polypeptide syndromes.

REFERENCES

1. Krejs G.J., Orci L., Canlow J.M., et al.: Somatostatinoma syndrome: Biochemical, morphologic and clinical features. *N. Engl. J. Med.* 301:285, 1979.
2. Baylin S.B.: Ectopic production of hormones and other proteins by tumors. *Hosp. Pract.* 10:117, 1975.

10 / Pheochromocytoma

MANAGEMENT PROBLEMS

The patient's complaints in pheochromocytoma include abnormality in the blood pressure and blood sugar. If the pheochromocytoma is unknown and persistent with low-grade symptoms, these are usually expressed as headache, sweating, palpitation and nervousness, pallor and coldness in the extremities and face, tremor, nausea, and fatigue. Severe psychological disorders can occur, with patients expressing feelings of depersonalization and an extremely anxious feeling of impending doom. Occasionally, the problem becomes a crisis for the patient and an urgent management problem for physicians when a paroxysm of hypertension, arrhythmias, and cardiovascular decompensation occurs.

The physician must be aware of these problems as expressed by the patient and be continually thinking about the possibility that the protean symptoms the patient relates may be based in the severe physiologic stress of excessive catecholamine secretion. The surgeon particularly must be conscious that an intraoperative crisis may be based in an undiagnosed case of pheochromocytoma and be prepared to deal with this emergency. With clinical suspicion of this diagnosis, screening tests are selected and diagnostic confirmation achieved through specific assays before tumor localization studies are carried out. During this diagnostic delay, the patient must be prepared and managed to prevent any life-threatening crises without interfering with biochemical testing. When the diagnosis is confirmed and the tumor is localized, operation may be performed safely in the well-prepared patient using specific techniques.

INTRODUCTION: THE TUMOR, HORMONES, AND SYNDROME

Pheochromocytoma may have replaced syphilis as the leading contender for Osler's designation "the great mimic." No two patients seem exactly alike. The classic presentation of hypertensive crises under stress and recognizable episodes that lead to diagnosis is actually uncommon. The author has treated patients who have been asymptomatic, normotensive, and even lacked biochemical abnormality on occasional urine and blood tests. On the other hand, unsuspected "pheos" have also caused dramatic, sometimes lethal, surprises. The atypical presentation is the rule.

In Figure 10–1 is shown the anesthesia chart of a patient with intraoperative cardiac arrests as her first diagnostic evidence of abnormality. Pheochromocytomas have also been called "physiologic bombs," underscoring the seriousness with which these cases must be treated. Even in the 1980s, a patient with an unsuspected pheochromocytoma who undergoes a stress-

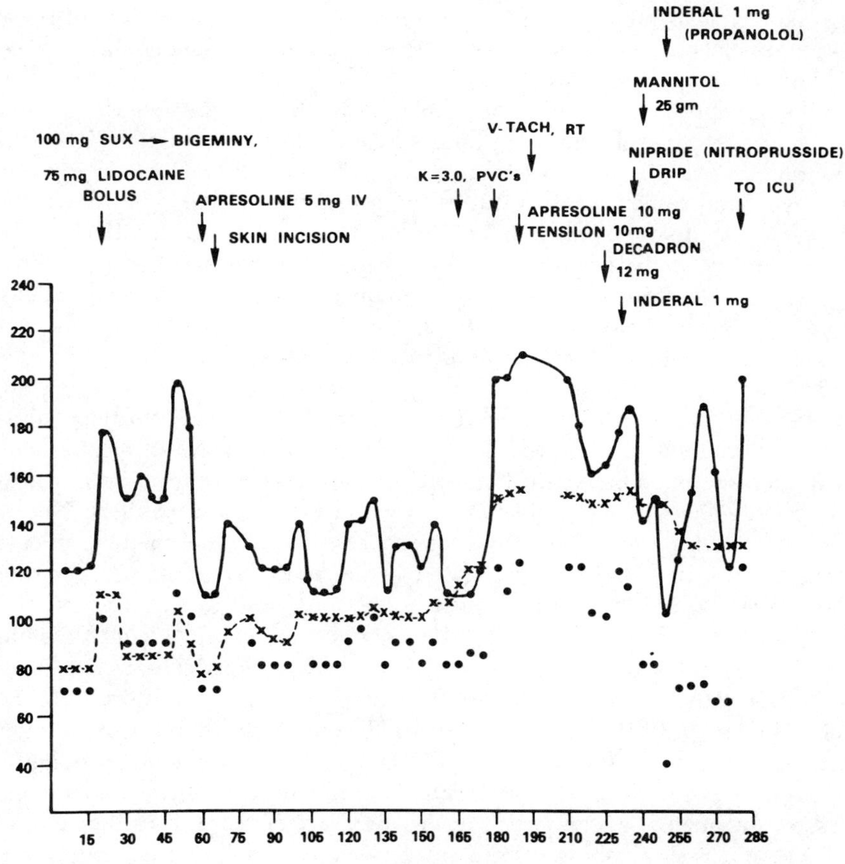

Fig 10–1.—The stormy operative course of a patient who underwent hip nailing while pheochromocytoma was unsuspected. It was later found that she had had similar intraoperative discovery of a prior pheochromocytoma 13 years earlier during hysterectomy.

ful situation such as childbirth, an accident, or an operation, has a 50% chance to come out alive unless the attending physicians recognize and appropriately manage the abnormality. There are few classic presentations for pheochromocytoma, and only a very sensitive index of suspicion will uncover the majority of the patients who have it. It is not an easy diagnosis to confirm, and screening nets a large number of patients who may have some of the features thought to be classic for pheochromocytoma but who do not have the disease. As an example, over the last several years, 35 patients per year on the average have been referred to the author for management of suspected pheochromocytoma, and from three to five of these patients per year are found to have the pheochromocytoma confirmed and treated.

Pheochromocytoma is a tumor that arises in chromaffin tissue, and chromaffin tissue is not anatomically limited to the adrenal medulla. The neuroendocrine APUD cells that migrate from the neural crest in embryology scatter along predictable distributions from the base of the skull, down the area of the sympathetic chain in cervical and thoracic areas, and throughout the retroperitoneum from diaphragm to bladder. Wherever these chromaffin cells are located, they share a common cytochemistry and argentaffin staining characteristics (hence the name pheochromocytoma) and the enzymatic metabolic machinery that allows them to take up amine precursors and decarboxylate them.[1] Any of these chromaffin cells can become neoplastic and give rise to a pheochromocytoma. Hence, pheochromocytoma is not an anatomical diagnosis that implies a specific organ of origin, such as the adrenal gland, but the tumor that may arise in quite different anatomical regions shares histologic identity and functional capability. Nearly the same clinical syndrome may originate from an adrenal pheochromocytoma as from the same tumor located in the neck, even though different names may be ascribed to this same neoplasm, based on its location. For the purposes of this discussion, the "glomus jugulare,"[2] "paraganglionoma," "organ of Zuckerkandl," "chemodectoma," "sympathicogonioma," and any other catecholamine-producing tumor of chromaffin-tissue origin produce similar pathophysiologic problems despite wide differences in their anatomical origin. Wherever this APUD neoplasm arises, it may retain its function of amine uptake, decarboxylation, and release of catecholamines. These catecholamines may exert a physiologic effect on the cardiovascular system, glucose metabolism, and nervous system, but if the tumor suddenly releases a large quantity of its stored catecholamines, pharmacologic effects may be seen. The typical pheochromocytoma that comes to diagnostic attention contains more catecholamine than the body can withstand if abruptly released into the circulation, and decompensation might occur.

The triggers for such abrupt release may be something that happens to the tumor, such as manipulation, massage, or compression by a particular body motion or external force; hemorrhagic necrosis and infarction as the tumor may outgrow its blood supply; or psychological or physiologic stimulation of the autonomic nervous system, such as exertion, pain, emotional distress, a transient decrease in blood pressure (e.g., the carotid sinus pressure of a tight collar), the Valsalva maneuver, or sexual arousal. Unintended provocative tests have uncovered pheochromocytoma in several patients treated by the author; glucagon is a useful hormone for GI endoscopy and radiography. Glucagon administration for barium enema, endoscopy, or facilitation of contrast CAT scanning is a potent stimulus to the release of catecholamine from a pheochromocytoma.[3]

Catecholamines that may be synthesized and released in chromaffin tissue include epinephrine, norepinephrine, and dopamine. The species of predominant catecholamine is determined by the enzyme concentration in the tissue of origin. The biogenic amines isolated from pheochromocytomas include the three catecholamines just mentioned and their metabolites, as well as 5-hydroxytryptamine (serotonin) and precursors. Catechol-o-methyltransferase (COMT) is the enzyme that is not present in very significant amounts in sympathetic nerves or in extra adrenal chromaffin tissue. Hence, such chromaffin tissue would release predominantly norepinephrine, lacking the methyltransferase COMT. The adrenal medulla, however, contains a large quantity of COMT activity, and, hence, catecholamine secretion from tumors of adrenal medullary origin may produce up to 80% of the catecholamines in the epinephrine species form. Epinephrine and norepinephrine are metabolized to the metanephrine and normetanephrine forms, and these excreted metabolites may give some clue as to the location of the tumor producing the excess catecholamines by the predominance of the catecholamine species in the blood or the metabolite of each species in the urine. This inference as to the origin of the excess catecholamines by this biochemical method is useful, since most other localization studies involve some manipulation of the sensitive and treacherous pheochromocytoma.

The physiologic half-life of the catecholamines injected into the circulation is very brief. Catecholamines are degraded, usually within 30 seconds of their entry into the bloodstream by the action of MAO. Any medications or competitive agents that inhibit the activity of MAO increase the circulating half-life of catecholamines and hence accentuate their physiologic activity.

The catecholamines represent classic neuroendocrine mediators. Typically, norepinephrine is considered a neurotransmitter, both in the CNS and in the autonomic nervous system, and rarely are sufficient quantities of this neurotransmitter circulating in the bloodstream to be considered a "hormone." Epinephrine is considered a hormone, since it is typically released from one location, circulates, and has its physiologic effect on a distant target site. These principles generally hold true under basal physiology, modulating blood flow and energy metabolism through a wide range of stress adaptation.[4] However, under severe stress, norepinephrine may be found in the circulation as a hormone, and, similarly, epinephrine may be found acting in the CNS as a neurotransmitter. But under the unusual circumstances of neoplastic transformation, excesses of circulating catecholamines can be seen in the circulation far in excess of values that can be secreted even in response to maximum stress. The "fight-or-flight adaptation" accomplished by these mediators in their dual roles as neural and humoral transmitters continues under these circumstances of hypersecretion, even if this stimulation is not purposeful. It is for this reason that pheochromocytoma can give rise to clinical symptoms that have been called the "panic syndrome."[5]

DIAGNOSIS: SCREENING, CONFIRMATION, AND LOCALIZATION

The presenting complaint of the patient with pheochromocytoma is so varied that specific examples from the author's experience will be cited, chiefly to show that each new patient seems unique. One young woman served as a softball coach, and once, while squatting on her haunches behind a batter she was coaching, she fell over on home plate with a paroxysmal attack. Another patient had no suspicious symptoms until a severe attack during the course of a glucagon-augmented barium enema performed for an unrelated indication. One young woman was being treated for "toxemia of pregnancy" when her blood pressure became uncontrollable, and a cesarean section was planned to relieve the preeclampsia. On application of the iodine abdominal preparation for the cesarean section, her blood pressure became unobtainable, and she was in pulmonary edema with marked mottling of the skin; for this reason, she was said to have a severe iodine sensitivity. Her diagnosis was confirmed when the stormy course of her cesarean section was complete, and the hypertension was not resolved following abdominal delivery. A young woman was having lunch in a restaurant across the street from my office when, following ingestion of some red wine and cheese, she became disoriented and had a pounding headache. A woman had had complaints of high blood pressure and high blood sugar, which she had discussed with eight different physicians with whom she had made appointments to show her diary of complaints, but remained undiagnosed. Then she observed that when she picked up the telephone from her low telephone stand by leaning over to the right, she had no problem, but whenever she turned her trunk to the left in leaning to pick up the phone with her left hand, she would fall over the phone, vomit, and require more than half an hour to recover from such an episode. One middle-aged man was referred by a psychiatrist who had been called in consultation to see him when the patient described a "forceful sensation in the pit of his stomach that pushed up through his chest to pull off his head." One of these attacks was observed, and the patient was proven to have an adrenal pheochromocytoma. A Spanish-speaking woman was admitted to the emergency room with a severe attack of chest pain which she could not further describe, and based on cardiography and blood pressure determinations, she was admitted to the coronary care unit for "cardiogenic shock"; her complaints and her cardiogram remained unchanged with the addition of abdominal pain, and a sonogram obtained to rule out suspected gallstones incidently revealed a large adrenal mass. A 60-year-old woman was admitted following hip fracture; 13 years before, she had had a kidney removed for a tumor. In the operating room for hip pinning, she had an unsettling anesthetic induction, but the operation proceeded, and during skin closure and reawakening she suffered ventricular tachycardia and cardiac arrest (see Fig 10–1). After a difficult resuscitation and stabilization, further information was received from the previous hospitalization that a similar incident had occurred 13 years previously during hysterectomy in which a large tumor had been found near the kidney, and both were removed. After adequate pretreatment, she underwent uneventful excision of a new pheochromocytoma in the opposite adrenal gland.

Many of these stories appear to be one-of-a-kind and would not be instructive except to point out that this atypicality seems to be the rule; the typical patient presentation may be during periods of unusual stress, and if the diagnosis is unsuspected, the mortality is forbidding. However, a number of patients present with baseline hypertension, with or without unusual symptoms of visceral, central, or autonomic nervous system abnormality, and with no history of paroxysms. Because of the very widespread prevalence of hypertension, the screening of "essential" hypertension would produce an unsatisfying yield of pheochromocytomas as a surgically curable etiology of hypertension. Among the approximately 20 million U.S. residents with hypertension, as many as 0.1% may harbor pheochromocytoma.[6] Although this figure would make it appear that pheochromocytoma is rare, it would more correctly be interpreted that it is rare to discover pheochromocytoma by screening patients with hypertension. Only by adding a physician's acuity in checking out unusual symptoms coupled with hypertension can the screening yield be increased. And the author has had occasion to operate on two individuals who were not and, as best it could be determined, never had been hypertensive! The point to be made in uncovering the diagnosis is that this physiologically malignant tumor is eminently worth finding, since it is curable in almost all cases. The loss of life from unknown or untreated pheochromocytoma has been estimated with a wide variety of conclusions; one overgenerous estimate that has been published[7] has been that 600 to 800 patients die annually in the United States of hypertension due to pheochromocytoma. In a smaller group of patients under unusual circumstances, somewhat greater precision can be drawn, and of patients with pheochromocytoma complicating pregnancy, maternal and fetal mortality has each been reported near 50%.[8] There are very good reasons for finding the tumor if we had an effective, reliable screening method that could be generally applied.

Some of the specific screening tests may be indicated by other tests not designed specifically to pick up pheochromocytoma as a diagnosis. For example, glucosuria or an elevated fasting blood glucose level may be present, or hemoconcentration may appear on review of the hematocrit. Electrocardiographic evidence can lead to pheochromocytoma within the differential diagnosis. Screening may be indicated for features that have nothing to do with the pheochromocytoma, but could be present with associated hyperparathyroidism, medullary thyroid carcinoma, or features of Cushing's syndrome. The screening studies thought to be specific for pheochromocytoma include the measurement of vanillylmandelic acid (VMA), which may be elevated in pheochromocytoma if the test is done correctly. The specificity of this test is problematic, since unrestricted diet, urine collection and storage, and sampling error may reveal normal VMA if collected from a patient during a quiescent period. Several drugs interfere with the measurement of VMA determinations, particularly the most commonly used antihypertensive agents. Furthermore, because of their nonspecificity, VMA determinations on urine may be supportive, but cannot confidently be relied upon to rule out a pheochromocytoma. Urine catecholamine assays may be somewhat more specific, and, as previously noted, may even give some indication of location of the primary tumor. Drawbacks to the determination of catecholamines and their breakdown products in the urine include the sensitivity of the assays to different patterns of activity, diet, drugs, and radiopaque media, and the cost if catecholamines, metanephrines, and VMA are collectively assayed. The assays for catecholamines are less widely available than the biochemical study of VMA. It is most helpful to have the patient one suspects of having episodes that may be pheochromocytoma paroxysms carry home with him a urine collection flask with the acid preservative already included, and instruct the patient to collect his urine for 24 hours following the paroxysm. If there is any indication in this urinary excretion of an increase in catecholamine, the patient may then return for an outpatient office procedure that is probably the single best test to confirm the presence of a pheochromocytoma.

In the author's experience, the best diagnostic confirmation comes from the measurement of serum catecholamines. This is done with a very specific technique that involves a special preparation of the patient. The patient is examined with the blood pressure taken supine, seated, and standing. He is then instructed to lie down comfortably in a bed in a specially-prepared room where he is not stimulated for 30 minutes following the examination. A venopuncture is carried out at the beginning of this period, and a "heparin lock" is placed with a scalp vein set. After 30 minutes of supine rest without excess stimulation, the syringe attached to the scalp vein is filled, the venous sample is transferred to a refrigerated special "cat-a-kit" tube, and this blood sample is centrifuged immediately and the serum frozen for radioimmunoassay of the catecholamine species. Bravo and coworkers[9] have found this serum catecholamine determination at basal conditions to be a highly reliable indicator of the presence of a pheochromocytoma, and the author concurs that false positive results in this experience are rare. There may be some individuals who have paroxysmal hypertension and positive urinary excretion studies that may have negative serum catecholamines on one or more occasions at rest, but the serum catecholamine determination has been the indication for progression from "noninvasive" to "invasive" localization studies on the author's protocol (Table 10–1).

A word of caution should be added regarding pharmacologic testing of pheochromocytoma patients. In general, pharmacologic tests for endocrine tumors should take the form of less dangerous "suppressive tests" than the sometimes hazardous "provocative tests." This is especially true for pheochromocytoma, but holds in other instances as well (see "Insulinoma" in

TABLE 10–1.—TUMOR LOCALIZATION STUDIES FOR PHEOCHROMOCYTOMAS

NONINVASIVE	INVASIVE
Analysis of catecholamine metabolites	Venous sampling
Abdominal x-ray and fluoroscopy	Venography
Sonography	Arteriography
CAT scan (caution: NO glucagon)	
IVP	
Iodocholesterol (or adrenal medullary) scanning	

chap. 6). Provocative tests are never indicated when the patient has marked hypertension, since the end point of provocation is a rise in the blood pressure. Not only is a provocative test dangerous if the patient has a sustained elevation in blood pressure, but the blood pressure variable may be dampened and the tests less conclusive. Furthermore, if a provocative test is employed (cold pressor stimulation, such as emersion of an extremity in ice water or administration of IV glucagon or of IV histamine), medications for immediately counteracting a positive further elevation in blood pressure should be available, mixed and ready for infusion. However, rapid overcorrection of the hypertensive effect of provocation may lower the blood pressure to less than normal levels, and this suppressor test to excess may be a second provocative stimulus when autonomic reflexes are triggered in a patient. As a general rule, provocative tests are never preferred to suppression tests in endocrine diagnosis, but when the provocative tests may be dangerous, they are contraindicated. In the case of pheochromocytoma, almost all provocative tests are obsolete. Screening of urinary metanephrine and plasma catecholamine determinations has an accuracy that has greatly diminished the utility of pressor tests.

A popular suppression test in the patient with sustained hypertension who might have a pheochromocytoma is the phentolamine test. In this evaluation, the patient's blood pressure is taken frequently, and an IV solution is maintained while saline controls and approximately 5 mg of phentolamine is run in. If a marked depression of blood pressure occurs following the transient α-adrenergic blocking drug, the result is called positive. When performing this study, pressors should be available for infusion, and usually noncatecholamine pressors such as angiotensin can be used if urinary catecholamine metabolites are being collected. As mentioned above, a very profound drop in the blood pressure can be a provocative test, and for both provocative and suppressive tests for pheochromocytoma, drugs should be available to counteract wide fluctuations in blood pressure, but also lidocaine, propranolol, α-blocking drugs, and volume expanders also should be ready for use. One provocative test that is mild, quite reliable, and avoids the need for pharmacologic injections is the "tilt test" in which a change in posture is the independent variable against which changes in blood pressure are compared.

If the patient has biochemical as well as clinical evidence of a pheochromocytoma, and the data from suppressive or provocative tests are convincing, even if the catecholamine assays have not yet been reported, a series of localization studies may be begun. In the author's experience, several of the noninvasive localization studies are done synchronously with the biochemical confirmation of the pheochromocytoma if suspicion is high, but preparation by adrenergic blockade is mandatory before invasive study. In practice, this means that the noninvasive localization studies are done at the time of urinary catecholamine collections, and after the serum catecholamine samplings, the patient begins receiving increasing dosages of α-adrenergic blocking drugs. By the time the optimal level of blockade has become effective, the results of the serum catecholamine studies are available, and preparations are made for invasive localization tests as an immediately preoperative measure.

Table 10–1 outlines the sequence of invasive vs. noninvasive localization studies. At the outset, it should be noted that "invasion" is a relative term, and does not imply only physical manipulation of the tumor. Psychological stress, pain experienced by the patient, and certain pharmacologic agents all can make a noninvasive study more seriously stressful than one of the invasive procedures. One very notable example of potent provocation by a presumably noninvasive study is the order for a CAT scan of the abdomen. Even if the physician ordering the study makes reference to the adrenal glands and the possibility that this patient has a pheochromocytoma, the specific instructions should still be relayed to the persons actually performing the study that *no glucagon* be used as is the routine for contrast-augmented CAT scanning. At least one patient in the author's experience suffered the only attack of her life in the CAT scanning suite, and experienced drenching sweats and crushing substernal chest pain with ECG changes following the demonstration of a left adrenal tumor before the glucagon was administered.[3] The distinction between invasive and noninvasive localization tests is made to point out that those patients undergoing invasive testing (that is, stressful by any of the criteria listed) must be pharmacologically prepared, monitored, and attended during such studies.

Patients do not need to run the gamut of the studies listed in Table 10–1, but only require sufficient studies to clarify two objectives: (1) location of the primary tumor and (2) screening of other chromaffin tissue sites outside the area of the prospective surgical field to exclude other anatomical sites of multiple tumors. For example, if a large tumor is apparent on sonography in one of the adrenal glands, yet the patient is excreting a considerable quantity of norepinephrine, one may wish to have information about anatomical sites other than the involved adrenal gland, such as that obtained by CAT scanning or arteriography. These studies in search of bilateral, ectopic, or multiple pheochromocytomas may be redundant proof of the localization of the first-noted tumor, but are particularly helpful if the search is conclusive outside the body cavity to be examined by operation. For example, abdominal exploration will not be able to test for cervical or thoracic ectopic sites.

It has previously been mentioned that the analysis of catecholamine metabolites may be helpful in inferring the site of a tumor to a very rough approximation, but these data are not conclusive, and further visualization would be required. The classic sequence for localization might include abdominal x-ray and fluoroscopy, coupled with intravenous pyelography. These data are helpful, particularly if nephrotomography is employed for examination of the suprarenal areas, and the bonus of this procedure is that "hypertensive pyelography" is obtained for further suggestions as to the etiology of hypertension in a patient not found to have a pheochromocytoma. However, the author's practice is to start with an ultrasound examination of the abdomen for noninvasive study. This test is truly noninvasive if the tumor is not massaged vigorously by the ultrasound probe and can reveal the tumor satisfactorily (Fig 10–2). However, resolution of sonography is usually not good enough to exclude other sites of chromaffin tissue abnormality. CAT scanning is currently much in vogue for noninvasive localization. It is true that resolution of the newer-generation scanners is excellent, but in the experience of the author false positive and false negative results have occurred that would cause a word of caution about the current enthusiasm for replacing arteriography with CAT scanning, and simply directing the operation at the CAT-demonstrated lesion, often from the posterior, retroperitoneal approach. The case has not yet been proven that CAT scanning can replace arteriography.[10] And furthermore, both localization stud-

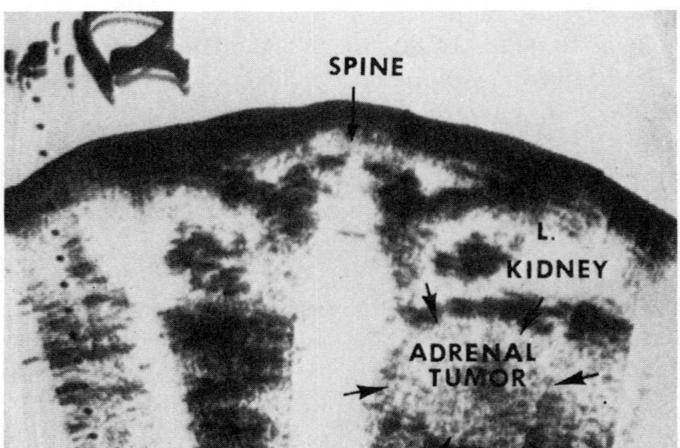

Fig 10–2.—Sonography is a successful noninvasive study for finding some pheochromocytomas, but resolution may not be high enough to exclude other sites.

ies and operation are directed at the definition of abnormalities in chromaffin system, and not simply at plucking out the demonstrated tumor.

Isotopic scanning is currently available in iodocholesterol adrenocortical visualization, but the radiation dosage and prolonged time course make this indirect test less valuable for the adrenal medulla than it is for small adrenal cortical tumors. Soon to be made available is a direct adrenal medullary scanning technique that is in clinical trial for patients, and may even have sufficient concentration in chromaffin tissue that therapeutic radiation may be delivered to metastatic pheochromocytoma.[11, 12]

Venous sampling is a very useful technique for localization of tissue that is secreting excess catecholamine, when the noninvasive studies cannot determine the source. Venous sampling, however, should not be interpreted as the same as adrenal venous cannulation and venography. The venous sampling technique referred to is that of "laminar flow" caval sampling for catecholamine determination at specified sites. By advancing the caval catheter to the superior cava, along the left lateral suprarenal and right lateral suprarenal inferior vena cava, and at the caval bifurcation, blood samples can be taken by gravity flow from the catheter, and assayed using the same technique as the catecholamine determination on the supine rest-

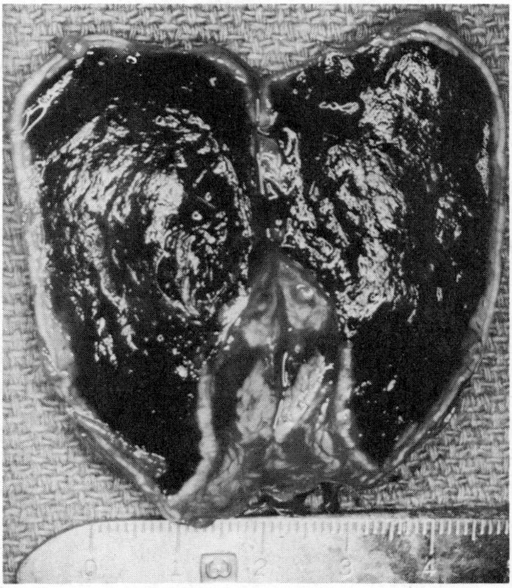

Fig 10–3.—A hazard of adrenal venography is that retrograde contrast injection may cause hemorrhage from the fragile veins and trigger a hypertensive crisis.

ing serum sample described above.[13] Caval sampling of this technique is minimally invasive, and can even be done on an outpatient basis without having full blockade with alphalytic drugs.

A considerable error is introduced by an attempt at venous sampling from adrenal glands. In the first place, the adrenal venous system is fragile, and retrograde injection of contrast material for venography can cause intra-adrenal medullary hemorrhage (Fig 10–3) and trigger a hypertensive crisis. But a second serious error is false localization information from an anatomically built-in sampling error.

Figure 10–4 shows an illustration of adrenal venous sampling and a remarkable step-up in the absolute serum catecholamine determinations sampled from the left adrenal region. This is an instance of false localization and illustrates the sampling error to which adrenal catheterization is prone. By manipulating the venous catheter through the left renal vein and up the central adrenal vein on the left, it is relatively easy to enter the adrenal effluent, and even to "wedge" the catheter and sample pure adrenal effluent. It is considerably more difficult to enter the right adrenal vein, which is very short and enters the right side of the inferior vena cava at

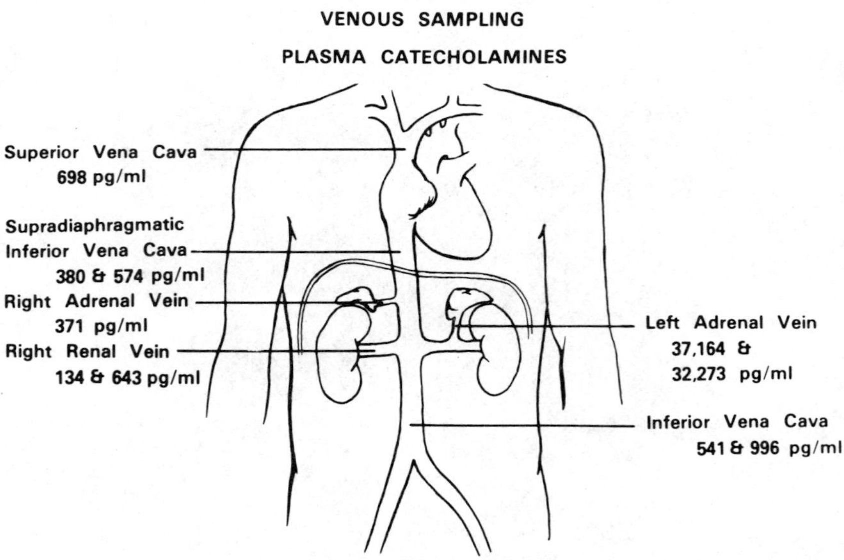

Fig 10–4.—A false localization, usually to the left adrenal gland, results when absolute catecholamine values are compared. This sampling error comes from the relative ease of cannulation of the left adrenal and pure adrenal effluent sampling, whereas the right adrenal catheter often samples caval admixtures.

right angles to the direction of the catheter. Often manipulation of this catheter is successful in instances later proven to be lumbar vein cannulation. When blood is drawn back from this catheter, frequently the sample obtained is an admixture of caval blood in the general adrenal region. Absolute values of catecholamine, therefore, comparing right and left, become in fact a measurement of the sampling error.

There are two ways around this problem of venous sampling. The first, already mentioned, was to perform gravity drainage of laminar flow samples, where the caval catheter is positioned in the "streaming" of the adrenal effluent from either side. This technique also avoids entry into and injury of the fragile adrenal veins. The second technique to avoid this error is never to trust absolute values for localization studies, but to use a ratio of the hormone under study with another hormone from the glands not involved in the neoplastic process. For example, in checking for the source of excess catecholamine release, one can study the catecholamine concentrations relative to cortisol. An example in which the absolute value would tend to suggest a localization to the side opposite the tumor location is illustrated in a comparison of hormone ratios (see Table 11–2).

Arteriography had remained the gold standard of pheochromocytoma localization tests, although newer techniques are eroding its dominant position, largely on the basis of additional safety for the patient with comparable resolution. Further supplanting of adrenal arteriography is expected

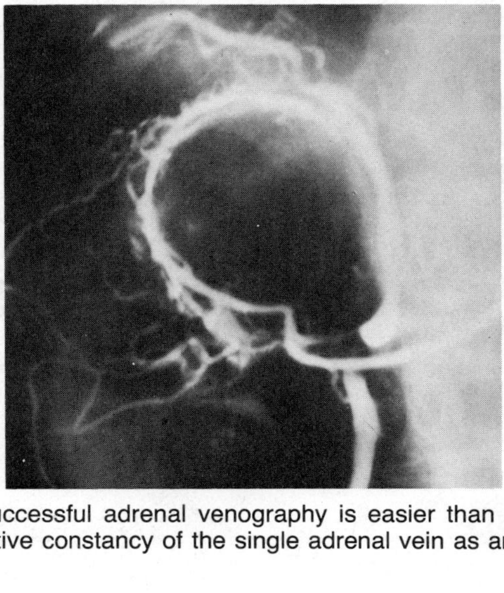

Fig 10–5.—Successful adrenal venography is easier than arteriography because of the relative constancy of the single adrenal vein as an anatomical hallmark.

when digital subtraction angiography becomes more widely available, achieving arteriographic resolution from an IV injection. Adrenal venography is much simpler than arteriography, however, with the relatively constant and single adrenal vein being a reliable anatomical landmark (Fig 10–5); the arterial supply to the adrenal gland is from generally three sources which are not easily catheterized, and may be variable. In other arteriographic searches for "tumor vascularity," it is the practice to inject epinephrine through the arteriographic catheter to constrict the smooth-muscle coats of normal arteries, leaving the less muscular neovascularity of the adenoma open for the contrast to shunt in a "tumor blush" (Fig 10–6). Injection of epinephrine into a patient who may already have excessive circulating pressors, and the stimulus to the tumor of both constrictor injection and contrast media injection provide a powerful provocative test. Venography and arteriography should *never* be carried out in the unprepared patient, should never be employed as outpatient localization procedures, and should usually be reserved as immediately preoperative studies. The preparation and monitoring required for these invasive studies are the same as those for operation (see the following section). These invasive studies are helpful in excluding other, not readily accessible anatomical sites before operative localization within one body cavity.

Final localization is carried out during operative exploration. When the acute infusion of blocking agents, such as nitroprusside, is discontinued,

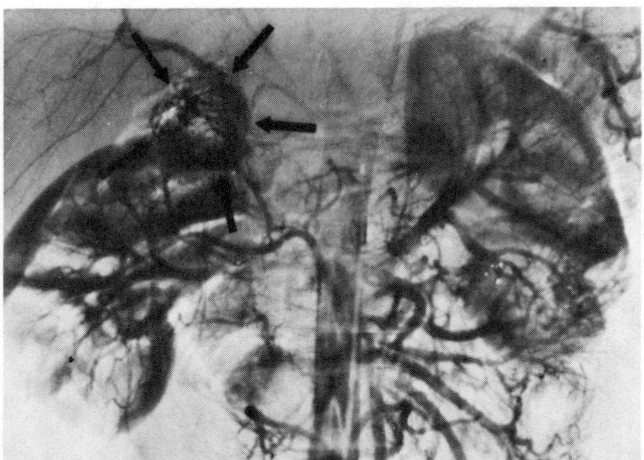

Fig 10–6.—Arteriography remains a highly discriminant localization method for pheochromocytoma, although it has hazards that require the same preparation as for operation.

following the removal of the tumor seen on noninvasive or invasive preoperative localization tests, a careful search of all other accessible sites of the chromaffin chain is carried out. As seen below in the intraoperative pressure monitoring records, multiple and ectopic pheochromocytomas may be uncovered by the physiologic pressor response to their manipulation.

PREOPERATIVE PREPARATION

Preoperative preparation of the pheochromocytoma patient is as important as the operative technique of tumor resection, and makes that operation safer. Although there are some differences of opinion as to whether all patients should undergo adrenergic blockade,[6] it is certainly safer for the patient to be so prepared, and this margin of safety can reduce emergencies in the patient's management and facilitate deliberate volume expansion and arrhythmia control. It is the author's practice to begin α-adrenergic blockade on an outpatient basis, while the serum catecholamine determinations are being assayed, and to continue increasing the alphalytic drug dosages over a period of gradual volume expansion. This is especially appropriate for the patient who may have hemoconcentration. A typical starting dose would be phenoxybenzamine given orally, 10 mg twice daily, while cautioning the patient against orthostatic hypotension and the other physiologic consequences of α-blockade. A blood volume determination is made at the beginning of α-blockade and immediately preoperatively. I have followed the indications reported by Harrison et al.[14] (Table 10–2) for the addition of β-blocking agents as the α-blockade increases. The most impor-

TABLE 10–2.—INDICATIONS FOR ADRENERGIC BLOCKADE IN PATIENTS WITH PHEOCHROMOCYTOMA*

Alphalytic agents (phentolamine, phenoxybenzamine)
Severe diastolic hypertension (> 200/130 mm Hg)
Frequent, severe paroxysmal attacks
Contracted plasma volume (hematocrit > 50%)
Use of betalytic agents
Betalytic agent (propranolol)
Tachycardia (pulse > 140/min)
Arrhythmia
Ventricular extrasystole
Pure epinephrine-secreting tumor

*Courtesy of Harrison T.S., et al.: *Surgical Disorders of the Adrenal Gland*. New York, Grune & Stratton, 1975, with modifications.

tant precaution with the use of adrenergic blockade is the sequence of agents employed. β-adrenergic blockade should *never* precede α-adrenergic blockade. It is a common practice currently to use propranolol as a first-line drug in the control of hypertension, and the patient whose hypertension is due to pheochromocytoma may develop pulmonary edema and heart failure given a β-adrenergic blockade while uncovered from the alpha effects of the catecholamine secretions. Most all patients receive α-adrenergic blockade, and many β-adrenergic blockade, but none receive propranolol without alphalytic protection.

A favored technique of the author has been the use of rapid-acting antihypertensive drugs given IV during crises or while the gradual oral buildup of the α-blocking reuptake-inhibiting drugs is taking place. The preferred agent for this protection has been nitroprusside,[15] particularly useful as the standby during invasive localization studies and intraoperative blood pressure control. Nitroprusside allows safe exploration by invasive study and by operation with a rapid metabolism when administration is stopped, allowing pressor responsiveness to return during exploration for other sites of additional chromaffin disease. Nitroprusside has also been useful in managing the crisis of heart failure in pheochromocytoma patients inadvertently given propranolol before the hypertension was known to be based in excess secretion of catecholamines.

Phentolamine, although it is a short-lived and rapidly acting alphalytic drug, is more expensive than phenoxybenzamine, which has a more prolonged duration of action. Phentolamine, however, has a cardiac depressant action of its own in accumulated dosage, and its short-term utility can be replaced with nitroprusside infusion. Propranolol is most often added only for the control of ventricular irritability and arrhythmias, and IV lidocaine is given for acute arrhythmia control as well. Propranolol should be used with caution in patients with Raynaud's phenomenon and in patients receiving digitalis or other predispositions to heart block.

A major component of preoperative and intraoperative management of the pheochromocytoma patient is volume replacement. The patient who has been under prolonged adrenergic stimulation often has severe blood volume contraction, and one of the major features of preoperative α-adrenergic blockade is the deliberate increase in capacitance preoperatively. Figure 10–7 illustrates the intraoperative record of a patient who received a light dose of phenoxybenzamine for the two weeks preceding operation. After removal of the tumor, with insignificant further blood loss, she exhibited very large "appetite" for blood transfusion, expanding the blood volume from the 50% of predicted values measured preoperatively. In some selected instances, part of the preoperative preparation includes a schedule

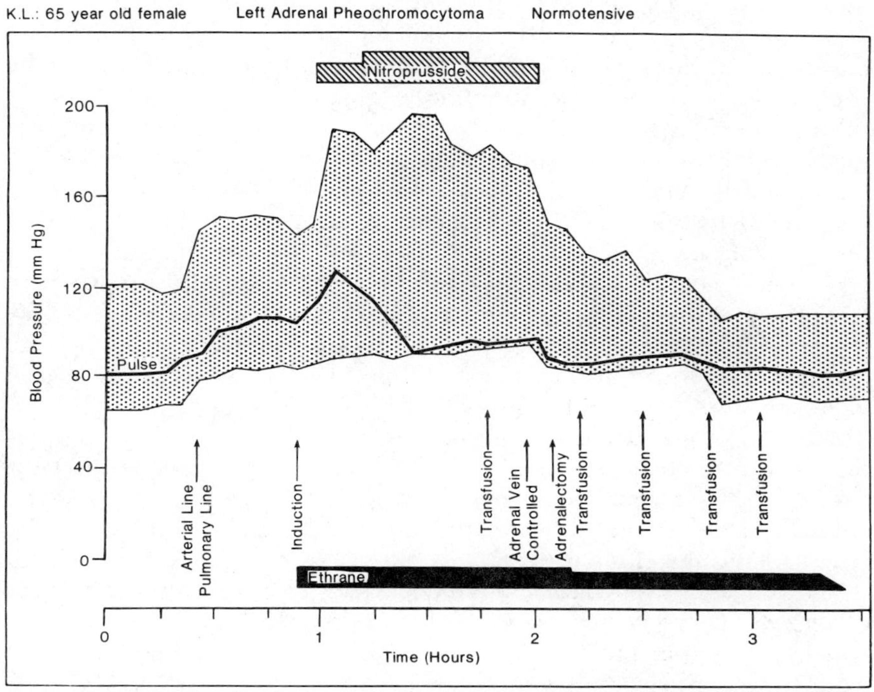

Fig 10–7.—Blood volume contraction is a major deficit in the pheochromocytoma patient who has not had adequate dilatation of capacitance by preoperative adrenergic blockade and volume expansion. The patient whose operating room record is shown received half a blood volume following tumor excision.

of steroid replacement, if bilateral pheochromocytoma is expected or if a previous adrenalectomy has been carried out. If possible, it is preferred that the corticosteroids are given immediately after the control of the pheochromocytoma.

ANESTHESIA MANAGEMENT

Close collaboration with the anesthesiologist and operating team requires preoperative consultation. In the author's experience, the standard practice has been to insert the monitoring lines the day before the operation and carry out the invasive localization tests, if indicated, with these monitoring systems in place and an anesthesia consultant available for administration of nitroprusside or other means of short-acting blood pressure control. The same monitoring systems remain in place as the patient goes from the immediately preoperative localization study to the operating room. An arterial line is a mandatory part of the operation for pheochromocytoma. Continuous display of the arterial blood pressure is a necessary component of the exploration and tumor resection. Cardiographic leads and central venous catheters also remain in place from the preoperative insertion, and premedication is given continuously from just before insertion of monitoring lines until the anesthesia is induced. The choice of premedication agents may be some tranquilizers to relieve anxiety on the patient's part, but morphine should be avoided because of its action in causing release of catecholamines and its histamine response, which can constitute a provocative test. The phenomenon of histamine release is also a contraindication to the use of some muscle relaxant agents; although pancuronium appears to be safe in this regard, a slight tachycardia and blood pressure elevation may follow its use.

A period of maximum risk and patient instability has usually been observed with intubation of the patient, and this period has been the most stressful for the patient and operating team alike. It can be made less hazardous by careful premedication and diligent attempts to avoid all unnecessary stimulation of the patient.

The choice of maintenance anesthetic agent for the patient with pheochromocytoma involves the advantages and disadvantages for each inhalation agent listed in Table 10–3. Methoxyflurane or balanced technique using fentanyl appear to be the inhalation anesthetic agents of choice, whereas some anesthetic agents are absolutely contraindicated (e.g., cyclopropane) or relatively contraindicated (e.g., halogenated agents) because of their myocardial sensitization potential. Adequate phenoxybenzamine preparation does not significantly reduce arrhythmias in pheochromocytoma pa-

TABLE 10–3.—ANESTHETIC AGENTS AND PHEOCHROMOCYTOMA

AGENT	ADVANTAGES AND DISADVANTAGES
Diethyl ether	+ Safe − Explosive
Methoxyflurane	+ Antiadrenergic − Nephrotoxicity
Nitrous oxide	+ Good analgesia − Some hypoxia
Halothane	+ Antiadrenergic − Myocardial sensitization
Enflurane	+ Good relaxation − Seizures with hypercarbia

tients, and propranolol in approximately 2-mg IV doses may be administered as necessary with lidocaine for control of arrhythmias.[16]

OPERATIVE TECHNIQUE

After the patient has had satisfactory induction and maintenance of general anesthesia and appears stable, careful preparation of the abdomen is done, avoiding vigorous scrubbing technique that may massage the tumor. The author prefers an abdominal transperitoneal approach in exploration for pheochromocytoma, since the operation is an exploration of the abdominal chromaffin chain, requiring careful inspection of the opposite adrenal, although all exploration and palpation of the abdomen are postponed until after the removal of the tumor localized by preoperative study. The focus of the operative approach is not on the tumor, but a swift and gentle dissection directed toward the control of the most important anatomical feature of the operation—the central adrenal vein.

The tumor contains dangerous, and potentially lethal, concentrations of catecholamines, even if the patient has undergone prolonged reuptake blockade. The primary objective in the operation is to obtain early control of the venous effluent from the tumor so as to exclude the pheochromocy-

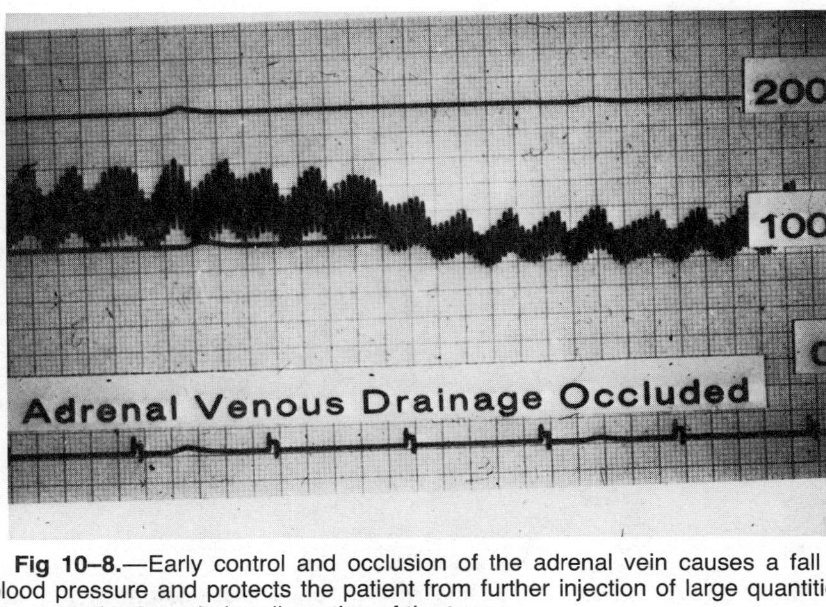

Fig 10–8.—Early control and occlusion of the adrenal vein causes a fall in blood pressure and protects the patient from further injection of large quantities of catecholamines during dissection of the tumor.

toma from access to the circulation. For a left adrenal tumor, this technique involves dissection down on the left renal vein and lateral progression until the central adrenal vein is encountered. Should the patient experience a crisis, the renal vein can be controlled, preventing injection of catecholamines into the circulation. As soon as possible, the left adrenal vein is exposed, and occluded with a vascular clamp or—the author's preference—with a large metal ligating clip. If the tumor is large, the adrenal vein is often similar in size to the renal vein. Occlusion of this very large-bore venous access route usually results in an immediate decrease in blood pressure (Fig 10–8). A similar technique can be carried out on the right side by dissecting down on the inferior vena cava and carefully exposing the right lateral border above the right renal vein.

With early venous occlusion and protection of the patient from adrenal effluent, nitroprusside or other agents administered during induction can be discontinued, and only then can exposure of the adrenal tumor and dissection of its arterial attachments be carried out. The process of tumor dissection is best described as "dissecting the patient away from the tumor." A technical feature that facilitates this dissection is the application of ligating clips around the margins of the tumor's attachments to the patient, and then, without manipulation of the tumor, cutting on the adrenal side

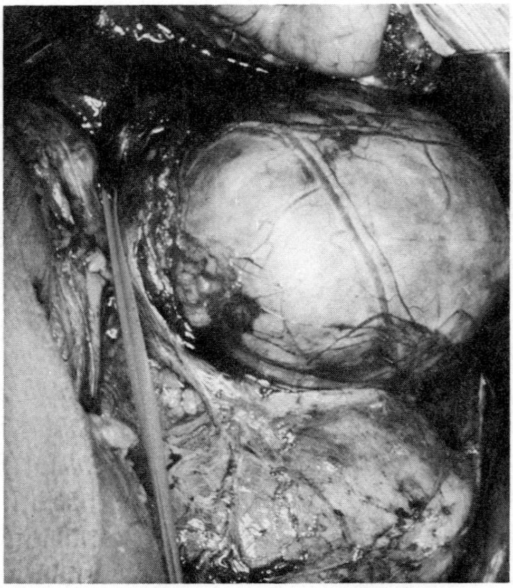

Fig 10–9.—After venous occlusion, the "patient is dissected away from the tumor" until the devascularized adrenal tumor can be excised.

of the clip. In this manner the suprarenal space is dissected until the devascularized adrenal and its tumor can be excised (Fig 10–9).

When the adrenal tumor has been excised, and a period of time has elapsed since the acute-acting antihypertensives have been discontinued, careful exploration is continued up and down the periaortic chain, with special attention to the opposite adrenal gland, the area of the organ of Zuckerkandl, and the dome of the bladder. If preoperative localization studies have suggested other suspicious sites, these are directly examined with palpation and massage while observing the arterial blood pressure.

An immediate fall in blood pressure following the excision of an adrenal tumor may be gratifying, but the operation is not complete until other intra-abdominal sites have been excluded. In a case of bilateral pheochromocytoma (Fig 10–10), an initial fall in blood pressure was followed by a hypertensive spike when the opposite adrenal was palpated. If operative exploration has been negative following the removal of the primary tumor and the general abdominal examination has found no other evidence of metastatic disease or other chromaffin tissue pressure hyperreactivity, provocative agents may be used intraoperatively. If the blood pressure has been stable and all evidence appears to indicate that the patient is free of

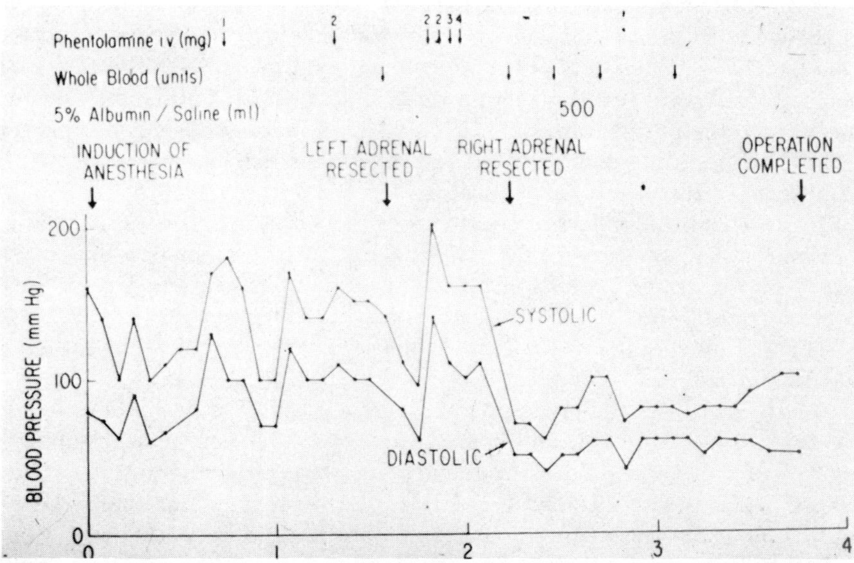

Fig 10–10.—Following an initial fall in blood pressure with excision of one adrenal gland, a rise in blood pressure signaled the presence of bilateral pheochromocytoma in this case of familial pheochromocytoma.

chromaffin tumor, 1 mg of IV glucagon can be administered to the patient while the abdomen remains open for exploration. A pressor response to this provocative stimulation may indicate a more diligent search in any of the ectopic sites within reach. The use of this provocative test and the blood pressure responsiveness intraoperatively is one of the reasons for employing short-acting blood pressure control medications and may be an additional reason, besides the toxicity of the drug, to prefer short-acting blocking agents over synthesis-blockade by such an agent as alpha-methyl-*p*-tyrosine.

Typically, the patient who has had indications of volume contraction begins to have dilatation immediately intraoperatively in the "catecholopenic" dilatation of the capacitance reservoirs. By arterial and central venous pressures, the patient receives transfusions to the extent necessary to fill up this volume deficit (see Fig 10–7).

POSTOPERATIVE CARE AND DRUG MANAGEMENT

Volume replacement is to be preferred over pressor administration for the management of the hypotension that may occur following excision of pheochromocytoma. A repeated blood volume determination can be made after the patient's hemodynamics have become stable, and the drugs used in preoperative preparation have been discontinued. If the patient has been found to have bilateral pheochromocytoma, or if a family history is suspected, serum and urine calcitonin determinations can be made following recovery in the postoperative period. If a strong index of suspicion suggests an MEA-II syndrome, calcitonin determinations can be made following stimulation with calcium or pentagastrin.

Over 90% of the pheochromocytomas removed at operation are benign, a diagnosis that comes more directly from operative examination than from histologic reporting. Patients may have recurrent pheochromocytoma, particularly those who have a familial history, or the recurrence may be a property of functioning metastases. Venous sampling by the caval catheter and "laminar flow" technique[13] may be helpful in locating these recurrent or new primary foci of functioning chromaffin tissue. Surgical attack at the functioning metastases or additional primary sites of new pheochromocytomas is a successful method of management, and drug therapy may take the form of sustained α-adrenergic blockade to relieve symptoms. Radiotherapy and chemotherapy for antitumor effect have been disappointing, and a combination of tumor reductive surgery and long-term phenoxybenzamine is a preferred method of management of persistent or metastatic pheochromocytoma. The most promising hope for specific treatment of metastatic pheochromocytoma is through the use of radioactive iodinated benzylguanidine.[12] The author has referred two patients with metastatic pheochromocytoma for therapeutic administration of treatment quantities of [^{131}I]*meta*-iodobenzylguanidine ([^{131}I]MIBG).

FOLLOW-UP AND SPECIAL CONSIDERATIONS

Special considerations for patients with pheochromocytoma in childhood, in pregnancy, at the "ectopic" extra-adrenal sites, and in familial kindreds should be acknowledged by the physician caring for such patients.

Cholelithiasis seems to be more common in the patient with pheochromocytoma, and other associated lesions are sometimes found in the neurocutaneous manifestations of neurofibromatosis or von Hippel-Lindau disease. Patients may also have the cutaneous manifestations of café-au-lait spots, often in the midline of the body on the dorsum of the back or neck. Some pheochromocytomas secrete ACTH, and Cushing's syndrome may be associated, and, in the author's experience, a number of patients with pheochromocytoma have had elevated calcitonin determinations which seem to be associated with the pheochromocytoma and not with medullary thyroid carcinoma.

Children with pheochromocytomas have convulsive disorders more frequently than do adults with the same diagnosis. Congenital cardiac defects may be present in some children with pheochromocytoma, and more children than adults have bilateral adrenal tumors. Bilateral adrenalectomy without preservation of the adrenal cortex requires careful glucocorticoid and mineralocorticoid replacement, particularly in growing children in whom the dosage must be periodically reappraised.

In one of the hereditary MEAs (see chap. 14) called MEA-IIb or MEA-III, a characteristic body habitus distinguishes these patients from those with Sipple's syndrome or MEA-II. The medullary thyroid carcinoma that is a component of this syndrome is particularly lethal, and early, intensive testing for thyroid abnormalities and the calcitonin-marker should be undertaken for total thyroidectomy early in the disease.

Pheochromocytoma that may originate in extra-abdominal sites, such as the glomus jugulare or chemodectoma, have similar functional properties with respect to their endocrine secretions, but have additional peculiar features, such as a propensity for venous invasion. Such an intravenous extension of this chromaffin neoplasm in no way constitutes a contraindication to operation intended for cure.[2] But preoperative awareness of this peculiar feature of these tumors allows the planning of an operation designed for distal control of the vein to prevent tumor embolus or subtotal resection.

The search for, localization of, and treatment of pheochromocytoma is a very gratifying challenge in endocrine surgery. Over 90% of these patients part company with their disease, which may be oncologically benign but is physiologically malignant. It is a very difficult task with a steep "learning curve" to recognize possible pheochromocytoma patients from among the myriad complaints which may be endocrinologically insignificant, but the search is well worth the effort, since pheochromocytoma patients are prime examples of the surgical endocrinology of a life-threatening, unseen tumor that is possible to be searched for, confirmed, found, and removed by endocrine surgical management.

REFERENCES

1. Geelhoed G.W.: Adrenal tumors, in Pilch Y., das Gupta T. (eds.): *Surgical Oncology*. New York, McGraw-Hill Book Co., 1981, chap. 31.
2. Chretien P.B., Engleman K., Hoye R.C., et al.: Surgical management of intravascular glomus jugulare tumors. *Am. J. Surg.* 122:740, 1971.
3. Geelhoed G.W.: CAT scan and catecholamines. *Surgery* 87:719, 1980.
4. Cryer P.H.: Physiology and pathophysiology of the human sympathoadrenal neuroendocrine system. *N. Engl. J. Med.* 303:436, 1980.
5. Scott H.W.: The panic syndrome: Pheochromocytoma, in Friesen S.R. (ed.): *Surgical Endocrinology*. Philadelphia, J.B. Lippincott Co., 1978, chap. 10.
6. Manger W., Gifford R.W.: *Pheochromocytoma*. New York, Springer-Verlag New York, 1977.
7. Graham J.B.: Pheochromocytoma and hypertension: An analysis of 207 cases. *Int. Abstr. Surg.* 92:105, 1951.
8. Geelhoed G.W.: Surgery of the endocrine glands in pregnancy, in Weingold A.B. (ed.): *Surgical Diseases During Pregnancy*. New York, Harper & Row, 1983, chap. 8.
9. Bravo E.L., Tarazi R.C., Gifford R.W., et al.: Circulating and urinary catecholamines in pheochromocytoma: Diagnostic and pathophysiologic implications. *N. Engl. J. Med.* 301:682, 1979.
10. Egdahl R.H.: CAT scanners and pheos: Diagnostic and policy issues. *N. Engl. J. Med.* 299:475, 1978.
11. Wieland D.M., Jiann-Long W., Brown L.E., et al.: Radiolabeled adrenergic neuron-blocking agents: Adrenomedullary imaging with (^{131}I) iodobenzylguanidine., *J. Nucl. Med.* 21:349, 1980.
12. Sisson J.C., Frager M.S., Valk T.W., et al.: Scintigraphic localization of pheochromocytoma. *N. Engl. J. Med.* 305:12, 1981.
13. Harrison T.S., Seaton J.F., Cerny J.C., et al.: Localization of pheochromocytoma by caval catheterization. *Arch. Surg.* 95:339, 1967.
14. Harrison T.S., Gann D.S., Edis A.J., et al.: *Surgical Disorders of the Adrenal Gland*. New York, Grune & Stratton, 1975.
15. Lipson A., Hsu I.H., Sherwin B., et al.: Nitroprusside in the management of a patient with pheochromocytoma. *J.A.M.A.* 239:427, 1978.
16. Oyama T.: *Anesthetic Management of Endocrine Disease*, New York, Springer-Verlag New York, 1973.

11 / Primary Aldosteronism

MANAGEMENT PROBLEMS

The patient with primary aldosteronism exhibits hypertension and may have muscle weakness, polyuria, and polydipsia. The patient may give further evidence of the sequelae of hypokalemia, but often primary aldosteronism is suspected in the patient whose symptoms are indistinguishable from those of other patients with "essential hypertension."

Problems for the physician's management include the initial suspicion and confirmation of aldosteronism and its differentiation between primary and secondary forms, and then the distinction of those patients with primary aldosteronism based in an adrenocortical adenoma rather than adrenocortical hyperplasia. These latter patients are selected for operation, and adenoma localization becomes a major task for the physician in studying the patient already confirmed in the diagnosis of primary aldosteronism.

INTRODUCTION: THE TUMOR, HORMONE, AND SYNDROME

Beginning with this chapter, a new class of endocrine syndromes is discussed, not directly dependent on APUD physiology. This group of adrenocortical syndromes is based in the lipid biochemistry of steroid hormones. The adrenal cortex and the gonads are of mesodermal origin, and their characteristic endocrine products are only indirectly linked with the APUD system.

One of these endocrine syndromes has a rather pure pathophysiology reflected in the hormone effect on mineral metabolism. In contrast to other hyperadrenocorticism, aldosteronism is *not* associated with somatic abnormalities. The mineralocorticoid aldosterone has an action that appears to be specific for the limited number of cells with aldosterone receptors that are capable of synthesizing specific protein activity induced by aldosterone.

As noted in Table 11–1, aldosterone was identified as the suspected mineralocorticoid in man shortly before Dr. Jerome Conn discovered a case in the University of Michigan's Psychiatric Hospital with findings that matched the theoretic effects postulated for an excess of this hormone. Some of the basic work that led to the understanding of aldosterone physiology and the

TABLE 11–1.—HISTORY OF PRIMARY ALDOSTERONISM

DATE	INVESTIGATOR	DISCOVERY
1943	Allbright	Postulated gluco- and mineralocorticoid, and an anabolic agent in adrenal
1947	Greep	Mineralocorticoid effect of deoxycorticosterone
1952	Simpson, Reichstein	Aldosterone identified
1955	Conn	Primary aldosteronism
1960	Kliman, Peterson	Double isotope dilution test of aldosterone
1965	Conn	Normokalemic aldosteronism
1975	Hunt, Biglieri	Posture test distinction of adenoma from bilateral hyperplasia
1977	Wilson	Aldosteronism with normal aldosterone excretion
1978	Zipser	Normotensive primary aldosteronism

eventual pathophysiology of primary aldosteronism came from the studies of acclimatization of army recruits brought from temperate latitudes to the tropics. Individuals so transported exhibit a remarkable adaptation in urinary excretion of sodium, and potassium, pH, and water balance. Exaggeration of this aldosterone physiology may lead to the pathology of hypertension, hypokalemia, and metabolic alkalosis.

Aldosterone is a renin-driven adrenocortical secretion under normal physiologic conditions, with important modulation during environmental changes. Renin is a juxtaglomerular hormone secreted by the kidney acting as a "volume sensor" (Fig 11–1). Renin release by the kidney occurs through stimulation of the juxtaglomerular apparatus acting as "stretch receptors" (the baroreceptor theory), stimulation of the macula densa acting as a "sodium sensor" (the sodium theory), or stimulation of the renal nerves that are seen to innervate the juxtaglomerular apparatus (the neural control hypothesis). The critical experiment to differentiate the major control mechanism is still awaited, but the sequence of events from the point of renin release is well-characterized. As noted in Figure 11–1, the angiotensin II (that results from the action of renin and another enzyme in the plasma) stimulates the outermost layer of the adrenal cortex to aldosterone synthesis and release. The action of this aldosterone in increasing sodium retention and volume expansion with an elevation in blood pressure quenches renin release from the kidney by any of the three theories just described. This feedback repression is very similar to the enzyme control systems seen in wholly intracellular systems[1].

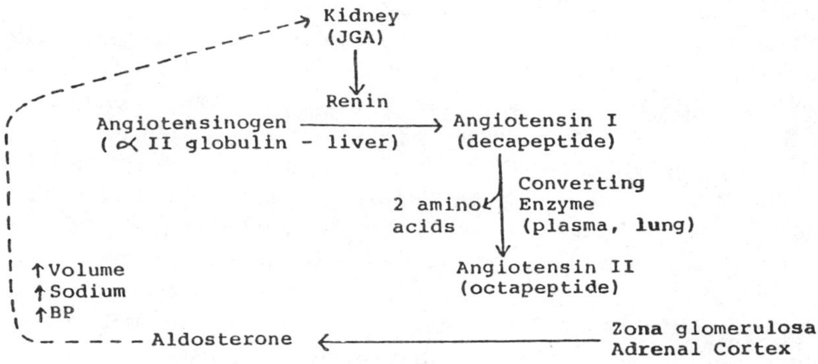

Fig 11–1.—The feedback control of aldosterone and its renin stimulus simulates wholly intracellular enzyme repression control systems.

In primary aldosteronism, this feedback of aldosterone on renin secretion [2] is ineffective in stopping the overproduction of aldosterone from the overactivity of one or both adrenal cortices. The sodium retention and potassium wasting and increased blood pressure that result are the features of the syndrome that bring the patient to a physician's attention. More subtle forms of this disorder may lack one or more of the classic features and later instances have been reported in which primary aldosteronism may exist in normokalemic individuals, and even those who are normotensive.

DIAGNOSIS: SCREENING, CONFIRMATION, AND LOCALIZATION

The hypertension of primary aldosteronism is usually of long duration and is mild; in contrast to the hypertension seen with pheochromocytoma, it usually produces no crisis and is not generally associated with the malignant hypertension that is followed by renal, cardiac, and CNS disorders. At the time of the discovery of the syndrome,[3] there was great enthusiasm for screening all patients with essential hypertension for this disorder because of a yield that was hoped to approximate 20% of the 30 million hypertensives in the United States. It is now known that far fewer than 1% of these patients will have primary aldosteronism as the source of their hypertension, and, much as with pheochromocytoma, the problem in management of this major public health problem resolves to "*whom* to screen?" Since this is mild and often medically manageable hypertension, a justifiable question might also be "why?" The answer to the latter is easier than the former, since primary aldosteronism represents a potentially curable form of hypertension and the restoration of normal physiologic balance in salt and water metabolism. But the question of screening is somewhat more complex, since few of the patients present with the classic features of hypokalemia that usually would be the strongest indication for screening. Some of these features include muscle weakness, cramps, fatigue, paralysis, and occasionally tetany in metabolic alkalosis. Low potassium also interferes in the function of insulin, and mild features of diabetes mellitus may appear. The hypokalemia and its symptoms may be spontaneous in its appearance in the patient, or it may appear immediately after the first use of thiazides to which primary aldosteronism patients are very sensitive. Since thiazide drugs are one of the first lines of defense in the management of hypertension, some primary aldosteronism patients are unmasked by their initial therapy. A similar hypokalemia may develop after salt loading, but this is less useful for a screening indication than is the application of thiazide diuretics, since most patients with newly discovered hypertension are given salt restricted diets by their physicians.

Among the initial screening tests that may be useful if a patient has spontaneous or thiazide-induced hypokalemia along with "essential hypertension" is the administration of a very short course of spironolactone; an immediate and remarkable decrease in blood pressure is not specific evidence for aldosteronism, but suggests further laboratory study.

The two steps in the laboratory diagnosis of primary aldosteronism are *confirmation* of aldosteronism and then *differentiation* of primary vs. secondary aldosteronism. Confirmation of aldosteronism may come by plasma assays of aldosterone, an aldosterone secretion rate, or urinary metabolite excretion. In some exceptional cases, aldosterone excretion may be normal despite hyperaldosteronism. A few of the diagnostic fine points that explain this abnormality include the direct inhibition of aldosterone synthesis by hypokalemia itself, and a differential of the glucuronide or other metabolites of aldosterone in the urine. Once having confirmed the excess secretion of aldosterone, the diagnosis is quite incomplete, since secondary aldosteronism (that is, renin-driven hypersecretion of the adrenal cortex) may result from a wide variety of stimuli, including renal artery stenosis, oral contraceptives, cirrhosis, nephrosis, congestive heart failure, and other, less common sources of an increased renin secretion. Therefore, plasma renin determination is done as the critical step in the differentiation of primary and secondary aldosteronism. It is important that plasma renin determination is made in the patient taking no diuretics, whose sodium intake is known on a plasma specimen taken when the patient is supine and resting, and also following upright posture and ambulation for several hours to reveal maximum renin levels. A near-zero upright plasma renin concentration in a patient with aldosterone excess is diagnostic of primary aldosteronism.

The further differentiation is required for indication of sugical therapy in distinction of an aldosterone-secreting adenoma of the cortex and a cortical hyperplasia—both of which may produce primary aldosteronism. Practically, during the workup with confirmation and differentiation laboratory tests, localization studies may also be carried out to distinguish mass lesions in the adrenal corex. However, an excellent physiologic test is the assay of recumbent- vs. upright-position plasma aldosterone.[4] Aldosterone decreases in patients with adenomas when the upright posture is assumed, whereas plasma aldosterone has increased when patients with hyperplasia have been upright. This physiologic test works in well with the assay of supine and upright renin determinations, and is helpful in differentiating between patients with cortical hyperplasia and with adenoma.

The next major hurdle in the diagnostic workup of primary aldosteronism involves localization of the suspected adrenal cortical adenoma. A review of the noninvasive techniques for the detection of mass lesions of the adrenal cortex is more hopeful for the future than it is currently—not yet reliable enough to dispense with the invasive studies. Sonography has been tried, but has not been helpful for the characteristically small (approximately 1.0 cm or less) benign aldosteronoma. As discrimination improves with gray-scale ultrasound combined with computed tomography, the resolution should be improved. The author does not share the uniform enthusiasm of some investigators who report that a CAT scan is all the localization required for operation on most patients with primary aldosteronism. The CAT scan is a good diagnostic test for the estimation of the size of the adrenal glands and can discern 1.0-cm adenomas, but the author has had mistaken lateralization on several "over-read" CAT scans, and for the small lesions, the resolution of CAT scanning has not replaced invasive contrast studies.

Iodocholesterol adrenal imaging utilizes radioiodine-tagged cholesterol several days before undergoing scintiscanning with the help of dexamethasone administration. The adenoma uptake of the isotope is early and strong, while contralateral gland visualization is delayed five to six days. In bilateral hyperplasia, there is no lateralizing dominant uptake, and dexamethasone suppresses radioactivity uptake for a prolonged period. The author has two reservations about the widespread applicability of iodocholesterol scanning for primary aldosteronism. The first is the high dosage of radiation to the patient undergoing scanning, and the second is misinterpretations of some of the cholesterol scans in his practice. In one instance, a phenomenon known as "unilateral micronodular hyperplasia" was diagnosed, and on this basis the patient was dissuaded from undergoing invasive testing, while hypertension and all other features of primary aldosteronism continued to be observed. Perhaps further experience using this technique on a large number of patients will contribute to its effectiveness.

Invasive studies have remained the key to the lateralization and surgical approach to correctable primary aldosteronism. Arteriography of the adrenal gland is made somewhat complex by the multiple arterial supply, but the high resolution makes arteriography of great value, identifying more than 75% of tumors larger than 7 mm in diameter (Fig 11–2). The diagnosis of hyperplasia cannot be comfortably made with angiography, although an enlarged adrenal gland is suggestive of the hyperplastic adrenal gland that may not contribute to evidence that the patient is an appropriate operative candidate. Adrenal arteriography in general is rapidly diminishing with the growing popularity of other tests that are more specific, such as iodocholesterol scanning, and tests that are easier to perform, such as CAT scanning or digital subtraction angiography. Adrenal venography, however, still has a considerable role in the definition of adrenal disease.

Venography is simpler than arteriography because of the single adrenal

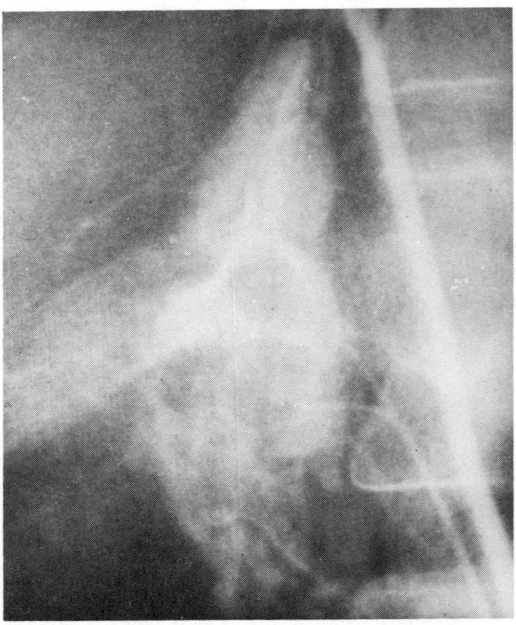

Fig 11–2.—Arteriography is an effective, high-resolution technique for aldosteronoma localization. For larger adenomas, arteriography may be replaced by CAT scanning.

vein that is the surgical and radiographic keystone of adrenal mass lesions. The right side is more difficult to catheterize than the adrenal gland on the left side of the body, and technical features of adrenal venography make it occasionally hazardous to the patient. Venography has very sizable advantages in that adenomas of 0.5 cm can be seen, simultaneous adrenal venous effluent measurements can be made, and lateralization of the corticosteroid ratios can direct the surgical approach. However, the procedure also has noteworthy disadvantages. The amount of retrograde pressure employed for effective visualization is nearly that which is effective in disrupting the delicate adrenal venous pattern, and extravasation may occur, not only obscuring the view of the adrenals, but destroying the glands as well. Hyperplasia cannot be adequately judged by adrenal venography. A major problem involves the interpretation of adrenal venous sampling data—frequently data on single steroids may suggest strong lateralization only because of a sampling error.

Adrenal venography (Fig 11–3) when positive is definitive in localization. However, caution in the interpretation of adrenal venous sampling must be urged, and the author would reject any absolute single steroid measurements that suggested lateralization, particularly to the left adrenal. As seen in Table 11–2, the sampling error possibility usually directs the attention

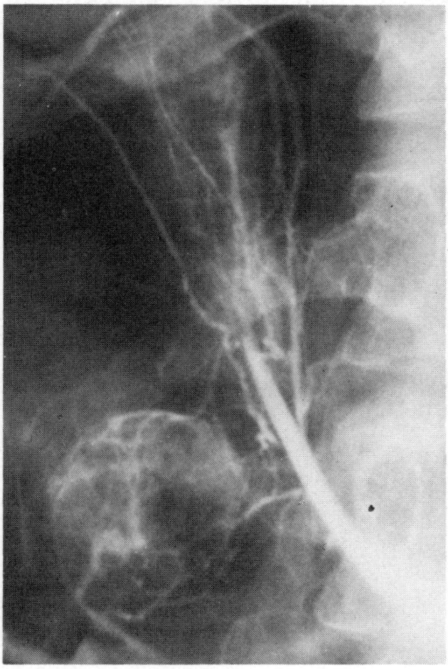

Fig 11–3.—Venography shows aldosteronomas even when they are quite small, and adds the bonus of venous blood sampling for determination of corticosteroid ratios.

TABLE 11–2.—EXAMPLE OF SAMPLING ERROR IN ADRENAL VENOUS SAMPLING*

RIGHT	LEFT	INTERPRETATION
Ratio: Aldosterone 1 :	8	Nonlocalizing
Ratio: Aldosterone 1 :	8	Lateralizing aldosteronoma
Ratio: Cortisol 1 :	48	on the *right*

*Case of a true step-up in which the left adrenal vein was cannulated and the right adrenal vein orifice approximated.

to the left adrenal gland. Since the left adrenal vein is easier to catheterize then the right, the sampling catheter slips up the left renal vein into the left adrenal vein, and usually represents pure adrenal effluent on the left. The right adrenal vein is short and comes off the cava at nearly a right angle, adjacent to lumbar veins which may also be catheterized. Sampling from this short vein may often yield mixed caval blood. An absolute left-to-right step-down results that is purely a matter of sampling concentrations (see Table 11–2).

Adrenal venous sampling for specific cortical adenomas should always use another steroid as a control, and the *ratio* then becomes the determining factor in a true step-up. As seen in the example in Table 11–2, a sampling error is shown in which a concentration value initially suggests much more aldosterone on the left than the right, giving a false localization to the left adrenal gland. When cortisol is also measured, the ratio of aldosterone-to-cortisol concentrations actually shows a step-up in the opposite direction, lateralizing the aldosteronoma to the *right*. Ratios, then, are far more reliable indicators of lateralization than are absolute concentrations from venous sampling data.

PREOPERATIVE PREPARATION

Localization studies have obviated bilateral exploration in all patients as was done initially[5] for patients with Conn's syndrome. The single most important feature of preoperative preparation is potassium repletion. Potassium supplementation is given at the rate of 6 to 8 gm of potassium chloride in the oral intake daily, but with simultaneous sodium restriction, since the patient with primary aldosteronism can waste great quantities of potassium supplementation if sodium is present in the diet in abundance. This competitive exchange occurs in both the GI tract and in the kidney, and potassium repletion is made possible by sodium restriction. A preferable alternative or adjunct to potassium supplementation and sodium restriction is the use of an aldosterone antagonist, spironolactone.

Spironolactone may be given at 400 mg/day for two weeks preoperatively to decrease the hypertension, aid in potassium repletion, and assist in correction of the metabolic alkalosis. Spironolactone may also suggest operative candidates and distinguish those who may not be effectively controlled by operation, since preparation at this dose is ineffective in some patients with bilateral adenomatous hyperplasia of the adrenals. The patient should be treated for hypertension without the thiazide diuretics that may have unmasked his hypokalemia, and the mild hypertension controlled with spironolactone or the addition of some other treatment form such as methyldopa.

ANESTHESIA MANAGEMENT

Once potassium repletion is satisfactory, the anesthetic management of the primary aldosteronism patient does not vary from the techniques used for any hypertensive patient. No corticosteroid pretreatment is necessary for the unilateral adrenal exploration, but if bilateral adrenal dissection is carried out, 100 mg of cortisol is suggested as a precaution against the transient cortical insufficiency from adrenal manipulation.[6] Curare is more prolonged in its effect in patients with hypokalemia and metabolic alkalosis, so succinylcholine is preferable to curare for muscle relaxation.

OPERATIVE TECHNIQUE

It is generally agreed that patients with proved adenomatous hyperplasia respond less well to surgical therapy than those with aldosterone-secreting adenomas. It is for this reason that the preoperative localization studies are so important, not only to distinguish primary from secondary aldosteronism—a determination made largely on the renin-aldosterone differential—but to exclude from operation those patients with less likelihood of benefit in cure of their hypertension and correction of their metabolic abnormalities. Patients with adenomas are nearly always cured by operation that is successful in finding and removing the focal source of aldosterone overproduction. Moreover, there is no urgency in the surgical correction of primary aldosteronism, since the hypertension is not acutely life-threatening. The operation should take place electively after fully adequate potassium repletion, and spironolactone blockade can be used for a temporizing measure for those patients who have other contraindications to operation. Long-term spironolactone therapy is the preferred treatment for bilateral hyperplasia of the zona glomerulosa, since bilateral adrenalectomy necessitates lifelong glucocorticoid and mineralocorticoid replacement as well as emergency measures for stress adaptation.

A second concern in the surgical management of primary aldosteronism based on aldosterone-secreting adenoma is the surgical approach. Bilateral adrenal exploration was carried out in the initial large series of these patients routinely, because of the small size of the adenomas and the lack of adequate resolution on most localization tests. A number of these small adenomas are found to occur bilaterally, and also it was thought indicated to perform bilateral adrenalectomy for bilateral hyperplasia, a controversial subject which has largely been resolved in favor of nonoperative treatment if the diagnosis can be made preoperatively.

The anterior transabdominal approach to adrenal masses is advisable if a cortical malignancy or large, nonfunctioning mass lesion is suspected, or if any evidence of medullary chromaffin disease is diagnosed preoperatively (see chap. 10). But for benign cortical lesions, especially if localized preoperatively, the retroperitoneal flank approach is preferred and is better tolerated by the patient. If the adrenal adenoma is localized preoperatively, a single incision and posterior approach to the retroperitoneal space through the bed of the 12th rib is the preferred approach. Bilateral adrenal exploration may still be indicated in some individuals by means of a simultaneous two-team approach (Fig 11–4). On at least one occasion, CAT scanning and invasive study indicated bilateral adenomas preoperatively and the bilateral approach was used for diagnosed bilateral adenomas, and not for exploratory indications. The left adrenal gland is the site of adenomas much more frequently than the right, approximately two thirds of the time. However, that is also approximately the ratio of adrenocortical mass in the normal individual, since the typical left adrenal gland weighs approximately 8 gm and the typical right gland weighs approximately 5 gm. If discrete adenomas are present bilaterally, the author attempts subtotal adrenalectomy with salvage of adrenal remnants, freeing the patient from steroid dependence. It is important to recognize the position of the central adrenal vein and preserve it if subtotal adrenalectomy is to be attempted. Subtotal adrenalectomy is a treatment for *adenoma,* however, and is not generally employed for hyperplasia either in the instance of primary aldosteronism or for Cushing's syndrome. Since the advent of CAT scanning, only two of my patients have undergone simultaneous bilateral retroperitoneal incision, and both of these patients were localized by preoperative invasive studies to both adrenal glands.

In the unilateral approach, the retroperitoneum is entered through the bed of the 12th rib, and the lumbodorsal fascia and transversalis fascia are incised to enter the retroperitoneum. At two points in the procedure, special care is taken to avoid entry into the pleural space by blunt dissection and reflection of the pleura before incision of the lower edge of the dia-

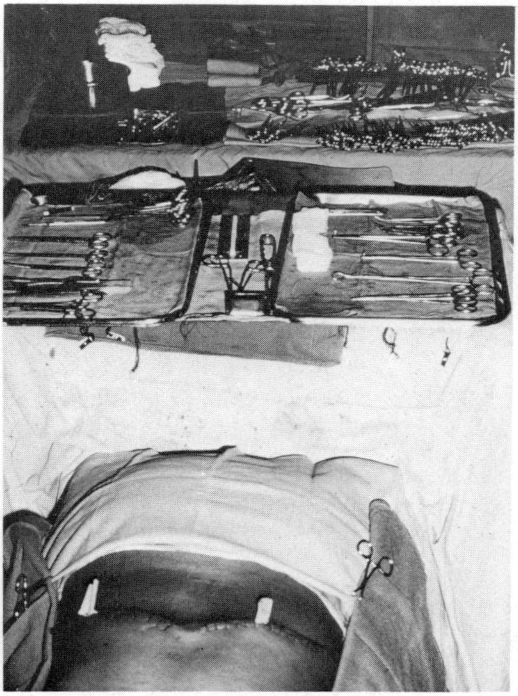

Fig 11–4.—Bilateral retroperitoneal approach is rarely used now if preoperative localization is successful in predicting a unilateral adenoma.

phragm and incision into the perirenal fascia. The adrenal gland is recognized on entry into the suprarenal space, and orientation by means of the central adrenal vein determines the extent of adrenalectomy. If a large adenoma is centrally placed or involves the central adrenal vein, total adrenalectomy is advised (Fig 11–5). If the adenoma is peripherally placed in an otherwise normal-appearing adrenal gland, subtotal adrenalectomy can be carried out.

A great advantage in the performance of adrenalectomy is the application of ligating clips.[7] In the event that a subtotal adrenalectomy is selected, a vascular clamp such as a Satinsky is placed along the midportion of the adrenal gland with care not to compromise the adrenal vein. The tumor-bearing adrenal cortex is then amputated, and the adrenal parenchyma is then oversewn with a vascular stitch, or more commonly in the author's practice, a line of ligating clips is used along the cut edge of the adrenal. While hemostasis is being achieved, attention is directed toward the kid-

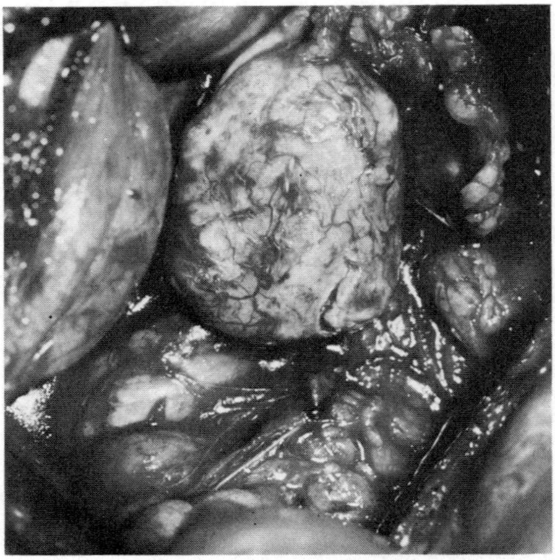

Fig 11–5.—The position and size of the aldosteronoma indicate subtotal or total adrenalectomy of the gland in which the tumor resides.

ney, and frequently a renal biopsy specimen is taken, particularly in hypertension of long standing. The renal biopsy is helpful for evidence of nephrosclerosis, and occasionally explains some residual hypertension postoperatively or may implicate some other etiology of the high blood pressure that may coexist with primary aldosteronism. A small drain is left as the fascial and muscular layers of the back are closed, and it is generally removed on the first postoperative day.

POSTOPERATIVE CARE AND DRUG MANAGEMENT

Immediately postoperative, the patient exhibits aldosteronopenia. This is marked by natriuresis, rapid repletion of potassium—usually up to a deficit of approximately 300 mEq net from the negative steady state to which the patient had become adjusted when the tumor was present. Urinary aldosterone frequently decreases to zero until residual adrenal cortex responds to the renin stimulus. The aldosterone decrease and the operative stress often result in a high renin state, which eventually stimulates the hypofunctional zona glomerulosa. The electrolyte abnormalities quickly resolve, but the hypertension frequently takes a matter of weeks before it becomes normal. There is no change in cortisol secretion nor requirement for administration in the event of a subtotal adrenalectomy, particularly if a single side approach has been carried out. Electrolytes and pH in blood studies are normalized before discharge of the patient, although blood pressure may not return to normal levels until the patient is ready for discharge from surgical follow-up in the outpatient clinic. During that interval, blood pressure regulation should take the form of antihypertensive drugs that do not include the thiazide diuretics or spironolactone. The author has followed up one patient whose blood pressure never completely normalized following removal of a large aldosterone-producing adenoma. Some component of essential hypertension may have been present in addition to primary aldosteronism, or some degree of glomerulosclerosis may have been a result of the earlier hypertension and a cause of the later, more manageable hypertension. At present the patient receives minimal drug therapy that easily regulates his blood pressure, and he has been asymptomatic since his electrolytes have normalized.

The aldosterone-producing tumor removed from a patient with primary aldosteronism (Fig 11–6) is rich in aldosterone and reflects the lipid content of the adrenal cortex, explaining the mineralocorticoid suppression that is seen postoperatively in aldosteronopenia. Recovery is generally rapid, particularly with the approach that does not involve entry into the peritoneum or pleural space. Interpretation of the renal biopsy is also helpful in predicting a return to completely normal blood pressure postoperatively.

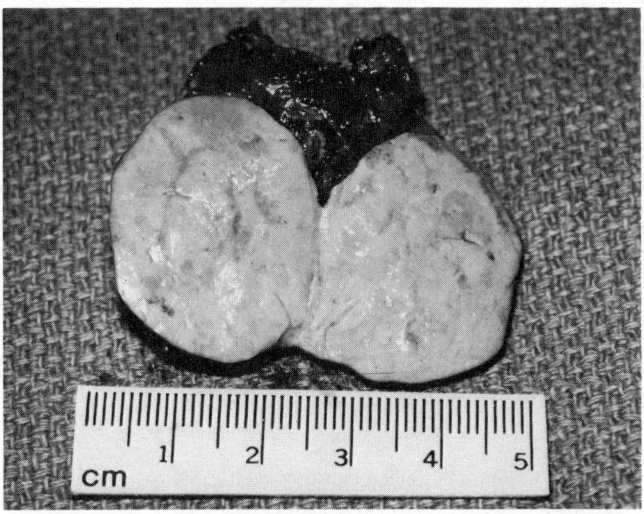

Fig 11–6.—On cut section, a large aldosteronoma shows the lipid steroid-rich tumor, accounting for the transient postoperative period of aldosteronopenia.

FOLLOW-UP AND SPECIAL CONSIDERATIONS

For the patient with bilateral micronodular hyperplasia, operation should be avoided if the diagnosis seems likely preoperatively. However, on some occasions, patients thought to have a localized aldosterone-secreting adenoma are found out to have no adenoma on exploration, but the adenomatous hyperplasia. Bilateral adrenalectomy is not advised in the treatment of this disorder, since medical management is preferred over adrenalectomy that would render the patient steroid-dependent. The cure rate for hypertension and electrolyte abnormalities is highly satisfactory for the patient with an adenoma, but although the electrolyte abnormalities may come back to normal quickly in the patient with hyperplasia, the blood pressure problem does not frequently resolve.

Occasionally, the patient with documented adenoma may have persistent hypertension for a protracted period. It is rare that this hypertension is on the basis of aldosteronism, since the patient's hyperaldosteronism is corrected by the removal of the adenoma. It is in these cases that the interpretation of the results of the renal biopsy studies and other data is helpful, since some of these patients may have other causes for their hypertension or essential hypertension made worse by the presence of the primary aldosteronism.

In summary, although primary aldosteronism is a rare cause of essential hypertension, it should be suspected particularly in patients who exhibit spontaneous or inducible hypokalemia. Confirmation of aldosteronism is by excess aldosterone secretion and excretion, but differentiation of primary aldosteronism is made on renin suppression. Localization studies help to differentiate adenomatous hyperplasia from aldosterone-secreting adenomas and indicate operative approach for the latter. With adequate preoperative potassium repletion in the confirmed primary aldosteronism patient with a localized adenoma, operation results in a long-term cure of the hypertension and associated metabolic abnormalities.

REFERENCES

1. Vander A.J., Geelhoed G.W.: Renin inhibition by angiotensin II. *Proc. Soc. Exp. Biol. Med.* 120:399, 1965.
2. Geelhoed G.W., Vander A.J.: The role of aldosterone in renin secretion. *Life Sci.* 6:525, 1967.
3. Conn J.W.: Part I: Painting background; Part II: Primary aldosteronism, a new clinical syndrome. *J. Lab. Clin. Med.* 45:3, 1955.
4. Hunt T.R., Schambelan M., Biglieri E.G.: Selection of patients and operative approach in primary aldosteronism. *Ann. Surg.* 182:353, 1975.

5. Nesbitt R.M. Primary aldosteronism: Its diagnosis and surgical management. *J. Urol*. 97:404, 1966.
6. Oyama T.: Aldosteronism, in *Anesthetic Management of Endocrine Disease*. New York, Springer-Verlag New York, 1973, p. 69.
7. Geelhoed G.W.: Surgical applications of radio-opaque ligating clips. *Contemp. Surg*. 11:9, 1977.

12 / Cushing's Syndrome

MANAGEMENT PROBLEMS

The patient with Cushing's syndrome has multiple problems that include a peculiar appearance and obesity, problems with control of blood pressure and blood sugar, weakness and muscle atrophy, hirsuitism, striae, plethora, acne, and easy bruisability with poor wound healing. Osteoporosis is often a problem, but is rarely recognized by the patient until the physician's examinations.

The problem for the physician in the management of Cushing's syndrome is in the recognition of the syndrome on the basis of endogenous hypercortisolism rather than on exogenous steroid administration. A major differentiation then takes place between those patients who have secondary (ACTH-driven) hypercortisolism on the basis of bilateral adrenocortical hyperplasia and those who have primary (autonomous adrenal) hypercortisolism, and whether the latter is due to unilateral benign or malignant tumor. If the Cushing's syndrome is on the basis of an adrenal tumor, and this tumor is benign, surgical cure of the Cushing's syndrome is very likely. For Cushing's Disease management methods will be quite different than for an operation designed for adrenal ablation; for adrenocortical carcinoma, operation may take place for attempt at cure, but more often palliation is achieved with specific drug management to help achieve comfort for the patient with disease that may spread widely.

INTRODUCTION: THE TUMOR, HORMONE, AND SYNDROME

The most frequent reason for the "cushingoid patient" is the exogenous administration of corticosteroid drugs. Whether the drugs come from a pharmacy or whether the same hormones or congeners are secreted by the patient, the syndrome that results is similar. The majority of patients with Cushing's syndrome from endogenous hypercortisolism have bilateral hyperplasia due to some excess ACTH or a polypeptide acting just like it in stimulating the adrenal cortex (see chap. 9, discussion of ectopic polypeptide hormones). This ACTH-driven cortisol excess is classic Cushing's Disease, either from pituitary basophilism as Cushing described it or from some paraneoplastic elaboration of ACTH-like hormones. About one fourth of all patients who have endogenous Cushing's syndrome have the syndrome based in an adrenal tumor as the autonomous source of the excess cortisol. Such patients are ten times more likely to be women than men and usually are in young adulthood. These patients experience severe disruption in their metabolism and changes in their lives during a period when they might be excellent rehabilitation candidates if the syndrome originates from a focal source that could be surgically correctable.

Almost all of the symptoms and signs of Cushing's syndrome relate to the glucocorticoid hypersecretion; some rare few of the patients with Cushing's Disease exhibit any evidence of pituitary mass effect (such as compression of cranial nerves), but some of these patients may also exhibit melanocyte-stimulating hormone (MSH) effect from ACTH excess. It is clear that the ACTH-driven Cushing's syndrome produces most of its pathology by adrenocortical stimulation, and ablation of the adrenal glands would relieve the patient of most of the signs and symptoms of Cushing's Disease. However, with the advent of specific techniques to ablate the primary source of pituitary-driven ACTH excess, endocrine surgeons are less often called upon to perform bilateral adrenalectomy if the primary problem resides elsewhere than the adrenal gland. There are also some candidates for "medical adrenalectomy" which may be used adjunctively with or in place of surgical adrenalectomy for the control of some of the features of the Cushing's syndrome. However, operation is among the most rapid and successful methods of control of hypercortisolism and is the treatment of choice for the Cushing's syndrome based in primary adrenal tumors. The diagnosis and the pathologic effect of the Cushing's syndrome is due to the overproduction of the hormones cortisol and, to a much lesser degree, corticosterone, which are essential in normal physiology in human glucocorticoid control of energy metabolism systems. Ablation of all cortisol secretion is not compatible with life unless a nearly physiologic replacement of this vital hormone is insured. It is not simply the excess of cortisol which makes the diagnosis of Cushing's syndrome. Chronic excess of the hormone does create Cushing's syndrome; however, absence of the hormone is a much more critical pathologic state. The pituitary-adrenal axis is the archetype of balanced endocrine control systems, and Cushing's syndrome is an imbalance in this system. Surgical therapy seeks to restore this balance rather than to eliminate the hormone responsible for the syndrome of hypercortisolism.

DIAGNOSIS: SCREENING, CONFIRMATION, AND LOCALIZATION

The diagnosis of Cushing's syndrome is *not* cortisol excess. The single diagnostic feature of Cushing's syndrome is the loss of the normal circadian physiologic pattern of ACTH and cortisol interdependency.

The patient to be screened for Cushing's syndrome does not always present with the fully developed classic picture of Cushing's syndrome, but may complain of muscle weakness, loss of energy, adult onset diabetes, susceptibility to infection, and unusual distributions of hair and fat, with skin changes. One of the most frequent complaints in my experience is an assortment of symptoms classified as mental illness—manic-depressive behavior, sleeplessness, and restlessness, with thought disturbances and hallucination, frequently bring these patients to psychiatric attention. Several young girls who were eventually found to have adrenocortical tumors have been referred for management following up to three years of behavioral and personality disturbances and over a year of psychiatric care before any stigmata of Cushing's syndrome appeared on physical diagnosis. One patient died in suicidal depression before the diagnosis of a potentially curable adenoma was made. Despite the severity of functional and metabolic disturbance, the primary source of the Cushing's syndrome is often difficult to determine. Although biochemical changes are suggestive, preoperative localization studies often suggest no abnormalities in mass, configuration, or total size or weight of pituitary or adrenal glands.

Sometimes cortisol determinations made in plasma or urine may be normal or even less than normal in the patient with features suggestive of Cushing's syndrome. However, the single best test is an AM and PM cortisol determination, and if the values are very closely similar, the patient exhibits loss of the circadian rhythm that is the diagnostic feature of Cushing's syndrome. The majority of patients have some elevation of cortisol, both in the plasma and in the excretion rate of metabolites recovered in the urine. ACTH levels may also be assayed, but are less reliable.

If the patient is found to have features suggestive of Cushing's syndrome and the two-point plasma cortisol determinations suggest a constant or elevated pattern of cortisol secretion, the patient is tested by an overnight low-dose (1 mg) dexamethasone suppression test. If the patient's cortisol measured in plasma is suppressed, it indicates the patient is having a normal response to ACTH suppression by the dexamethasone. This evidence indicates that the adrenal glands are following the signals sent by the hypothalamus by way of the pituitary. If no suppression is seen and the urinary cortisol metabolites are also suggestive, a tentative diagnosis of Cushing's syndrome is made, and the patient receives high-dose dexamethasone

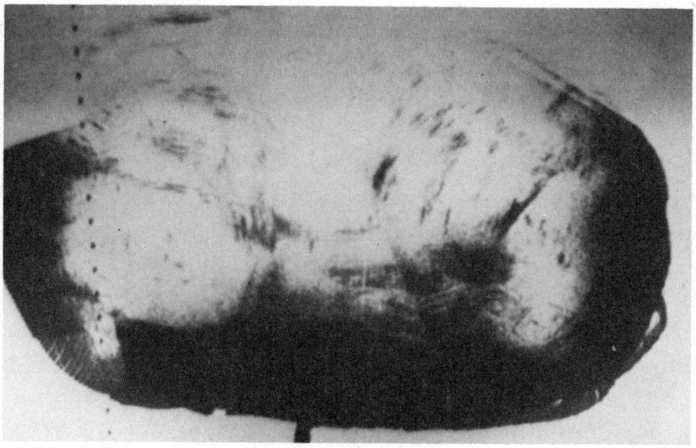

Fig 12–1.—Sonography located this very large adrenocortical adenoma in a young girl with primary complaints of psychiatric disturbance and minimal recent changes in skin and hair texture.

(8 mg/day for three days). If there is no suppression at this level of dexamethasone administration, either the adrenal gland is autonomously making too much cortisol, or it is not the pituitary that is producing the ACTH-like stimulation to the adrenal. In the absence of any other evidence of a nonendocrine primary tumor, the patient can undergo noninvasive study of the adrenal and pituitary glands by sonography and x-ray study (Figs 12–1 and 12–2). The single most valuable noninvasive localizing study is the

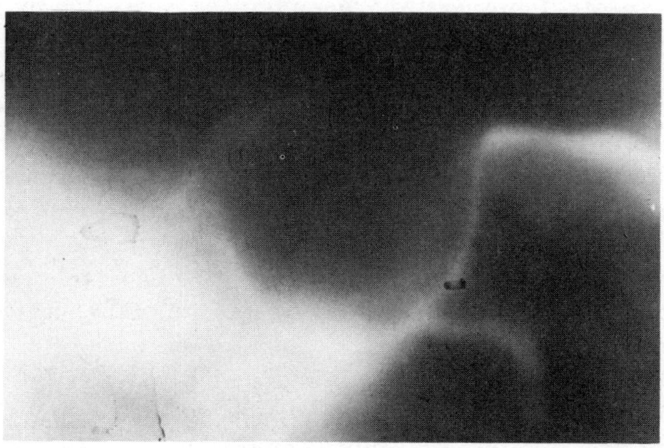

Fig 12–2.—Pituitary primary lesion was suggested by sellar tomography in a patient with florid features of Cushing's syndrome and severe depression.

CAT scan for defining adrenal enlargement. The radioiodinated cholesterol scintiscan should also be lateralizing in the patients with adrenocortical tumor, but the greater time course required by this study over CAT scanning probably contraindicates it, despite the advantages of its specificity for steroid-producing tumors. One of the disadvantages of CAT scanning is its nonspecific identification of enlargements that may not be functionally significant. In the patients who have Cushing's syndrome, the identification of an enlarged adrenal gland is often presumptive evidence of an adrenal tumor as the cause of the Cushing's syndrome, but as discussed in chapter 13, this is not always the case with adrenal masses that are imaged by nonspecific radiologic techniques. If the noninvasive tests are inconclusive, arteriographic and venographic studies are appropriate. Venography has the additional bonus of venous sampling for lateralization, but the same precaution for sampling error as seen in Table 11–2 applies in dealing with the products of the zona fasciculata of the adrenal cortex—namely, it is the ratio of corticosteroid hormones rather than their absolute concentrations that is important in the lateralization of adrenal tumors.

PREOPERATIVE PREPARATION

The objective of therapy for hypercortisolism is to remove any functional tumor responsible for the Cushing's syndrome that is not easily controlled medically. A second objective is the reduction of the hypercortisolism toward normal, and even more important, the preservation of normal pituitary and adrenal function and a return to circadian balance. A third objective is to accomplish these primary goals without permanent dependence on hormone substitution therapy. Operation makes possible the realization of some of these objectives for some forms of Cushing's syndrome. For Cushing's Disease this may take the form of a microdissection of the anterior pituitary through the transsphenoidal approach. An alternative to this surgical pituitary ablation is radiation therapy by means of Bragg peak ionizing radiation either for suppression or destruction of the anterior pituitary. Other forms of control may employ operation for control of paraendocrine tumors or the use of adrenocorticolytic drugs.

For the application of any of these primary treatment programs, the patient must be carefully prepared with consideration of the metabolic abnormalities that have resulted from the Cushing's syndrome.

Preoperative preparation focuses on reducing blood pressure, correcting potassium deficit, and conventional therapy for heart failure and for symptomatic diabetes. Corticosteroid pretreatment is not necessary, since uncontrolled hypercortisolism is the reason for the metabolic imbalance in the first place. Not until the day of the operation should consideration be given to steroid replacement, and a prolonged high-dose treatment regimen may merely switch the patient from endogenous hypercortisolism to an iatrogenic form of the same disease. Stress values of cortisol can be given to the patient in a dose of 100 mg IV during the operation and 100 mg IV postoperatively, supplemented with 200 mg of cortisone acetate intramuscularly for the first three postoperative days. No mineralocorticoid is necessary until approximately a week postoperatively, and the patient can take in the necessary mineralocorticoid replacement as fluorocortisone acetate at approximately 0.05 mg/day. The nutritional requirements for these patients are considered preoperatively, and the healing deficits are recognized, but nutrition cannot be pushed by total parenteral nutrition without balancing it with exogenous insulin administration as well.

ANESTHESIA MANAGEMENT

Obesity and muscle weakness cause interference with the inhalation or injection of many of the fat-soluble anesthetic agents and their distribution. The short neck, buffalo hump, and potential for pathologic fracture cause the patient to be fragile from the standpoint of hyperextension, intubation, and positioning on the operating room table, and the thin skin with easy bruisability is also considered when the patient has padding placed over pressure points for prolonged periods of immobilization. The blood pressure may be sensitive to changes in position, but any prolonged hypotension that occurs during the course of an operation in a patient with Cushing's syndrome should be treated with corticosteroid administration if no other obvious cause is recognized immediately.

Ether, cyclopropane, and halothane anesthesia stimulates adrenocortical activity in man, whereas methoxyflurane and enflurane (Ethrane) anesthesia do not.[1] Thiopental decreases plasma cortisol and is the anesthetic agent of choice for induction. Many approaches for adrenalectomy require muscle relaxants to be administered in the balance of anesthetic agents employed.

OPERATIVE TECHNIQUE

A transabdominal approach is recommended from anterior or flank position if an adrenocortical carcinoma is strongly suspected (Fig 12–3) or if a paraneoplastic tumor is the primary indication for operation, with an incidental attention directed to the adrenal glands as a target of the ACTH-like ectopic stimulation from the primary tumor. These indications are in the minority, however, and for most benign cortical disease, the retroperi-

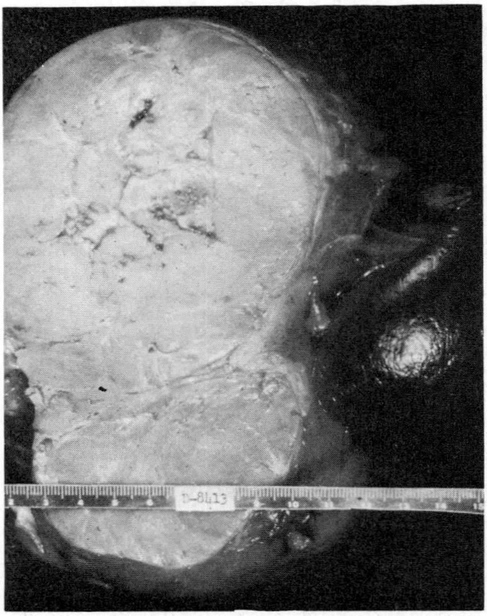

Fig 12–3.—A large adrenocortical carcinoma encountered in a patient with Cushing's syndrome was resected with the adjacent spleen by means of a flank approach.

toneal approach is recommended. Bilateral total adrenalectomy is still a treatment for Cushing's Disease, although not the treatment of choice in those who are amenable to direct pituitary attack with microsurgical dissection. However, bilateral adrenalectomy is successful in immediately reducing cortisol levels, even if the price paid for the rapid control is the lifelong dependency on administered steroids. Subtotal adrenalectomy for Cushing's syndrome that is driven by ACTH from the pituitary or an ectopic source is doomed to recurrence,[2] however, and this operation is to be discouraged.

For unilateral disease that has been localized preoperatively and is suspected to be a benign adenoma, approach is much the same as for unilateral primary aldosteronism as described in chapter 11. The approach through the bed of the 12th rib and the careful entry into the suprarenal space, avoiding pleura or peritoneum, allows a very good exposure to the entire retroperitoneum, including retropleural extension. In dealing with larger adenomas, careful dissection must be carried to the adherent plane between adrenal tumor and vena cava, and inspection for direct invasion of these structures may suggest that the preoperative diagnosis may be changed to adenocarcinoma if any of these features are encountered.

In closure of the wound, consideration is given to the poor healing exhibited by patients with Cushing's syndrome, and the integrity of the closure is insured by a longer retention of the sutures and careful tissue handling.

POSTOPERATIVE CARE AND DRUG MANAGEMENT

As mentioned initially, with Cushing's syndrome the findings in the adrenal gland may be surprising, since the normalcy of some of the adrenal glands that give rise to Cushing's syndrome is their most remarkable feature (Fig 12–4). However, some of the adenomas that are discrete and confidently diagnosed as benign, well-contained adrenal neoplasms must be very cautiously interpreted in projecting the prognosis for the patient and family. One such very benign-appearing neoplasm seen in sonography was suspicious only because of its size, but had no other histologic characteristics of

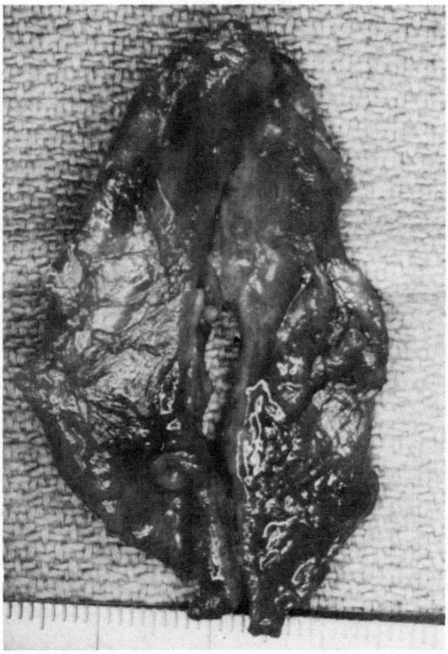

Fig 12–4.—The adrenal gland in some instances of Cushing's syndrome is remarkable in its nearly normal appearance despite proved hyperactivity. This adrenal gland in section is not more than twice normal weight, but the patient's hypercortisolism was severe.

malignancy (see Fig 12–1). Within three years of its resection, however, the patient exhibited a recurrence of Cushing's syndrome and thoracotomy-proven metastases in both lung fields.

Some methods of drug treatment can manage recurrent or persistent hypercortisolism by the interference with the adrenal synthesis of steroids or chemotherapeutic destruction of the adrenals in modified attempt at controlled medical adrenalectomy. Metyrapone or aminoglutethimide may be given to inhibit steroid biosynthesis. Sometimes the temporary reduction in steroids from these treatments is useful in preoperative preparation, but long-term management with these agents is not successful. O,p′-DDD (ortho-*p*-prime DDD) is a chlorophenothane (DDT) derivative that has been successful as a specific therapy for adrenocortical carcinoma.[3] To be effective, however, o,p′-DDD must be administered in toxic doses that have GI and CNS side effects, so this form of cytotoxic therapy is not useful as a "medical adrenalectomy" more benign than operative adrenalectomy.

Of special note in the postoperative period, in the author's experience, is the high incidence of thromboembolism in patients operated on for Cushing's syndrome. One death has occurred from postoperative pulmonary embolism in a patient otherwise recovering following adrenalectomy, and several persons have developed deep venous thrombosis; in the author's practice, patients with Cushing's syndrome are at high risk for thromboembolism and are given low-dose prophylactic heparin subcutaneously.

FOLLOW-UP AND SPECIAL CONSIDERATIONS

Patients who have had bilateral total adrenalectomy are obviously in need of steroid replacement. The schedule for this replacement regimen is shown in chapter 15 (see Table 15–2). For those who have undergone unilateral adrenalectomy or removal of adenoma in the adrenal or pituitary area for benign Cushing's syndrome the prognosis is excellent. Metabolic change is seen within the first postoperative weeks, and the patient's appearance resolves toward normal in several months. Two major sequelae that should be looked for after treatment of Cushing's syndrome are recurrence of the disease and Nelson's syndrome.

Nelson's syndrome is a problem that may occur in patients treated by bilateral adrenalectomy in whom a pituitary adenoma was responsible for their Cushing's Disease. The patient with Nelson's syndrome becomes hyperpigmented from the MSH effect of excess ACTH, and Cushing's syndrome may recur at these high ACTH stimulation levels. The most serious consequence of Nelson's syndrome is the progressive enlargement of the pituitary tumor to the point where "field cuts" develop from optic nerve compression.

For patients who have been adequately treated and followed up five to ten years postoperatively, the recurrence rate of Cushing's syndrome approximates 10%.[4] However, the patients who have adrenocortical carcinoma are excluded from this group of five- to ten-year follow-up by virtue of the grave prognosis of this diagnosis. Most of the adrenocortical cancer patients have disease that disseminates through the bloodstream, with pulmonary metastases that limit life despite availability of such drugs as o,p'-DDD and its usefulness is limited by its toxicity. One of the features that make this recurrent disease less manageable is the recurrent Cushing's syndrome that comes along with the tumor in those metastases that are functional, causing metabolic imbalance in the patient as well as the tumor cachexia of the progressive neoplasm.

REFERENCES

1. Oyama T.: Cushing's syndrome, in *Anesthetic Management of Endocrine Disease*. New York, Springer-Verlag New York, 1973, p. 63.
2. Egdahl R.H.: Surgery of the adrenal gland. *N. Engl. J. Med.* 278:939, 1968.
3. Fisher D.A., Parios T.C., Melby J.C.: Therapy of adrenocortical cancer with o,p'-DDD. *J. Clin. Endocrinol. Metab.* 25:218, 1963.
4. Hunt T.K., Tyrrell J.B.: Cushing's syndrome: Hypercortisolism, in Friesen S.R. (ed.): *Surgical Endocrinology: Clinical Syndromes*. Philadelphia, J.B. Lippincott, 1978, chap. 20.

13 / Adrenal Mass Lesions

MANAGEMENT PROBLEMS

The patient with an adrenal mass does not usually exhibit any abnormality early in the course of the disease. In fact, if nonfunctional, the mass may be silent and appear only as an incidental finding during examination for some other abnormality. The fear of the unknown nature of these space-occupying masses becomes an indication for further investigation. Unlike the thyroid nodule, the adrenal mass is hidden in one of the most "silent" areas of the body and does not cause patient complaints and impaired function of adjacent structures until it is of huge proportion. But like the thyroid mass, the presence of the mass itself is the worrisome feature that the patient must then have investigated and explained by the physician.

The problem for the physician's management is the differential diagnosis of the mass and the distinction of the significant from the anatomically trivial abnormalities. This can often be done with confidence only by resection of these mass lesions, and special features about them must be known before this undertaking.

INTRODUCTION

Existence of the adrenal mass lesion of unknown nature is a relatively recent phenomenon, largely a product of our improved noninvasive diagnostic techniques. As discussed in chapter 3, the thyroid mass lesion is often endocrinologically insignificant, but happens to occur in a gland that is endocrinologically active, and it may displace some of that function. Moreover, the thyroid gland is easily palpable, whereas the normal adrenal gland is not. Even when very large adrenal masses are present, they may remain undiagnosed. But, as has occurred with thyroid scanning, which discloses nonpalpable mass lesions even in this readily accessible organ in the neck, the availability of sonography and computerized tomography has revealed a number of mass lesions in the abdomen that must then be explained if they originate in the adrenal gland. Several of these adrenal masses have been known before, when they achieved such a size as to be palpable or to displace other organs—for example, depressing the kidney on IVP.

Some adrenal lesions may also calcify, and these masses are then found on standard x-ray examination of the abdomen. But the adrenal gland is even more obscure than the pancreas as a site in which hidden nodules can develop to appreciable size without detection. Their appearance in either the pancreas or adrenal glands requires an explanation, since several serious abnormalities can result, especially with masses that are nonfunctional, without endocrine evidence of their activity. Nonfunctioning adrenal tumors are even more suspicious than those that may give rise to glucocorticoid or mineralocorticoid excess, feminization, or masculinization. One of the possibilities that must be ruled out is that the unknown adrenal mass may represent one of these potentially functional tumors that has become undifferentiated to the point that no coherent endocrine messengers are being secreted. These tumors, with a serious prognosis, are mixed in with a number of adrenal mass lesions that must be further identified.[1]

Mass lesions of the adrenal gland can be classified by their etiology: they may represent hemorrhage, adrenal cyst, hyperplasia, adenoma, carcinoma, or metastases from neoplasms at other sites in the body.

Adrenal hemorrhage may be the result of trauma, such as the specific trauma of diagnostic catheterization and venography (see Fig 10–3). Adrenal hemorrhage can occur as a result of trauma or inflammation, injuring both cortex and medulla because of their common arterial supply and single venous drainage. Meningococcemia may cause hemorrhagic destruction of both adrenal glands in the Waterhouse-Friderichsen syndrome. The lethal nature of this disorder is coupled with the stress of the infectious disease and the failure of the adrenal cortex in the acute addisonian crisis brought on by the hemorrhagic ablation of the adrenal glands.

Adrenal cyst may present as adrenal tumor.[2] Besides diagnostic confusion with other adrenal tumors, in the author's experience an adrenal cyst has caused renovascular hypertension, and has been reported to cause symptoms when ruptured during blunt trauma.[3] The appearance of a very large adrenal cyst at operation is seen in Figure 13–1. This huge cyst had displaced the kidney and was actually thought to be an intrahepatic mass, but approached posteriorly without entry into pleura or peritoneum, the fluid content of this cyst was aspirated, and the cyst was completely excised without even the sacrifice of the major portion of the adrenal gland on the affected side.

Hyperplasia is not often thought of as a mass lesion occurring in the adrenal gland. However, adrenocortical hyperplasia (Fig 13–2) can cause a very enlarged adrenal gland—in this case of a treated adrenogenital syndrome, the mass of the adrenal had displaced the kidney on IVP. Adrenal adenomas are the subject of the preceding two chapters as known by their

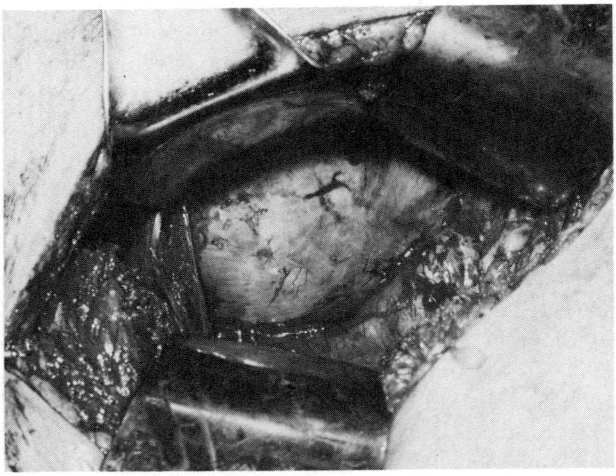

Fig 13–1.—Appearance of a large adrenal cyst at operation. After aspiration of the fluid contents, a subtotal resection of the adrenal with complete extirpation of the cyst was possible without entry into pleura or peritoneum from this posterior approach.

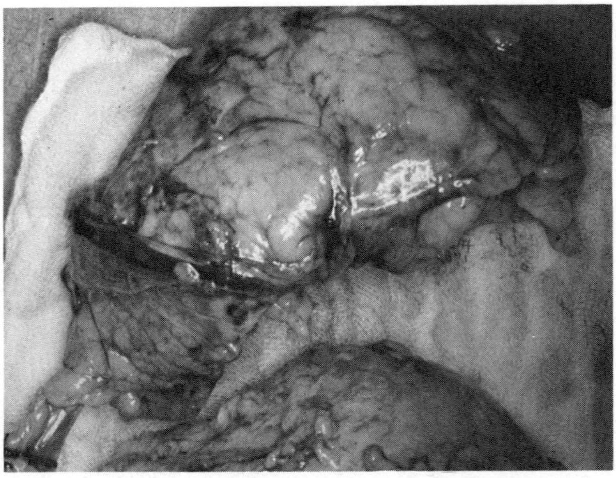

Fig 13–2.—Adrenal hyperplasia may be a cause of adrenal mass, as in this incidentally encountered mass in a patient with treated adrenogenital syndrome.

functional characteristics. But not all adenomas are functional, and an occasional nonfunctioning adenoma is encountered at operation performed for other purposes or is discovered by x-ray examination as an incidental finding.[4]

A neoplasm that is not of adrenal origin may metastasize to the adrenal glands, a condition frequently seen with bronchogenic carcinoma. This site of metastasis is not significant with respect to the cure of the bronchogenic carcinoma, but it may frequently displace and destroy functioning adrenal tissue and cause death from acute addisonian crisis in a patient whose adrenals are ablated by such metastatic disease. However, the adrenal gland may also be the site of origin of nonadrenal tumors. Two examples follow in which the adrenal gland was the primary site of a nonendocrine tumor.

A young radiology technician volunteered for a sonographic study as part of an exhibit on the normal ultrasonic examination of the female abdomen, when an abnormality was noted on the sonogram (Fig 13–3). CAT scanning confirmed the presence and solid consistency of this mass, first indicated on sonography, although tests for adrenal functional abnormalities were unrevealing. As seen in Figure 13–4, at exploration a lymphoproliferative neoplasm was discovered involving, but not originating in, the adrenal parenchyma.

The rapid development of a very large mass that was not associated with endocrine abnormality became apparent to a 50-year-old man who presented to his physician with a large, solid mass filling the right abdomen and flank. A CAT scan (Fig 13–5) suggested the adrenal location of this solid mass. Surgical approach by means of a thoracoabdominal incision

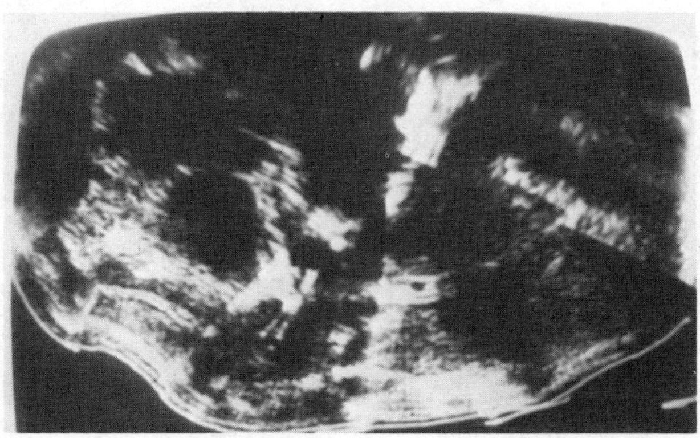

Fig 13–3.—An incidental finding on this "normal abdominal sonogram" was a large adrenal mass in an asymptomatic volunteer.

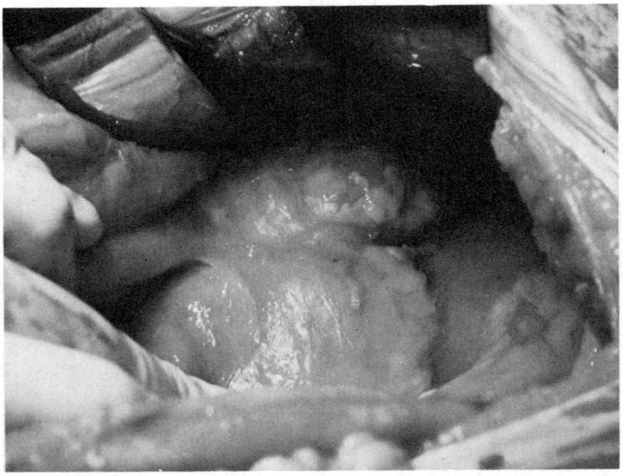

Fig 13–4.—Exploration uncovered a lymphoproliferative neoplasm in the adrenal area, involving, but not originating in, adrenal parenchyma.

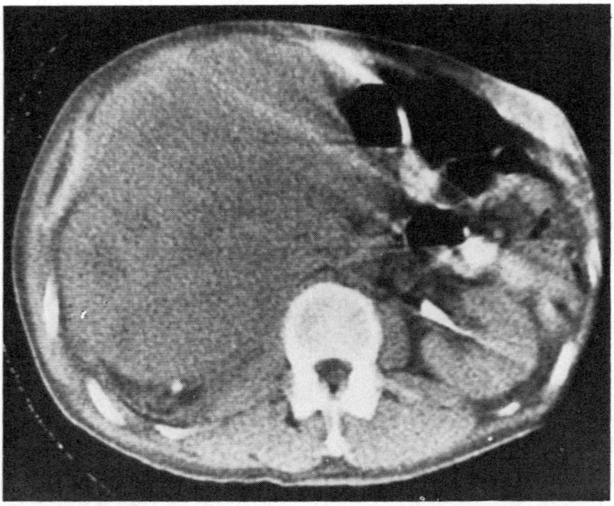

Fig 13–5.—CAT scan confirmed presence of a very large retroperitoneal mass palpable in the abdomen and flank of a patient without endocrinologic abnormality.

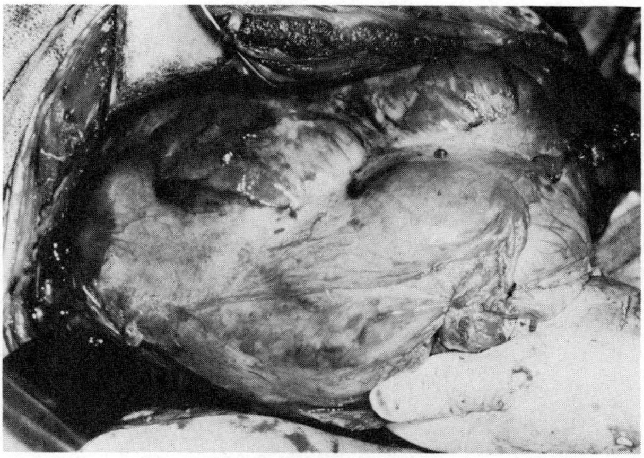

Fig 13–6.—Thoracoabdominal resection of the huge nonfunctioning tumor later revealed it to be a malignant fibrous histiocytoma originating in the right adrenal gland.

through the bed of the 10th rib made possible the resection of a massive tumor later proved to be a malignant fibrous histiocytoma of the right adrenal gland (Fig 13–6).

DIAGNOSIS

Adrenal mass lesions of this mixed group can cause relative and absolute adrenal insufficiency. All patients who have such adrenal mass findings should be tested for normal baseline and stress levels of corticosteroid function, particularly before invasive diagnostic maneuver or operative resection. The diagnostic techniques employed for space-occupying masses in the retroperitoneum are discussed in chapter 10 and summarized in Table 10–1. It should be pointed out that iodocholesterol scanning for adrenal mass lesion should be looked upon as a positive test for a "hot" nodule (Fig 13–7); a suppression of iodocholesterol uptake on the side of the mass may simply indicate the displacement of the active cholesterol-incorporating cortex of the biochemically active adrenal parenchyma by nonfunctioning tissue or fluid that does not take up the iodocholesterol.

PREOPERATIVE PREPARATION

Besides the mass localization studies that in many cases first indicated the presence of the suspicious adrenal lesion, preoperative preparation should

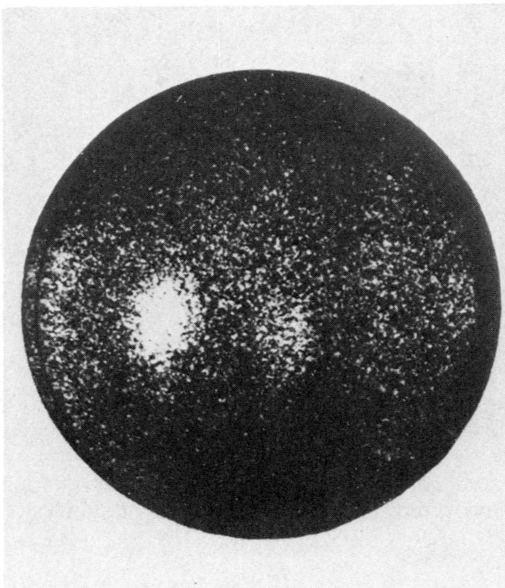

Fig 13–7.—Iodocholesterol adrenal scan 12 days after the radioisotope administration showed a "hot" concentration in one adrenal. Suppression of the opposite adrenal cannot be inferred if much of the adrenal cortex on the affected side is displaced by nonfunctioning fluid or tissue mass.

include tests for both normal and stress functional capability of the adrenal cortex. These function tests should precede all invasive localization studies to avoid the unprotected activation of a presumed nonfunctioning tumor. These tests include metabolite excretion, suppression tests, and, possibly for this indication more than is generally true for adrenal lesions with hyperfunctional baselines, provocative tests.

ANESTHETIC MANAGEMENT

For nonfunctional tumors in the patient being operated on who has normal adrenocortical function, no special anesthetic precautions are taken. However, any operation on the adrenal gland must be presumed to have a higher risk of an addisonian insufficiency from displacement of normal adrenal cortical parenchyma.

OPERATIVE TECHNIQUE

As seen in Figure 13–1, a successful operative approach can be carried out through a retroperitoneal exploration without entry into peritoneum or pleura for those lesions confidently predicted preoperatively to be benign, nonfunctioning cortical lesions. The patient tolerates this approach very well and can be discharged within three days in most cases.

For those lesions in which a primary adrenal carcinoma or metastatic carcinoma is suspected, an approach that will encounter the primary focus of the disease as well as access to regional areas of spread is recommended. This is often the anterior or the flank approach, allowing an extension into the abdomen.

An important feature of large adrenocortical mass lesions is their propensity for venous invasion.[5] Preoperative venography is especially helpful in making this diagnosis and in suggesting an operative approach for early distal venous control, both to prevent tumor embolization and to avoid subtotal resection of the primary tumor without consideration of its intravenous extension.

POSTOPERATIVE CARE AND DRUG MANAGEMENT

The postoperative considerations are largely dependent on the pathology report and the findings uncovered during the operation. Postoperative care may vary from the simplest observation for the patient with a successful cyst resection to the specific drug therapy for primary or metastatic carcinoma to the adrenal gland.

FOLLOW-UP AND SPECIAL CONSIDERATIONS

For adrenal masses and tumors that extend from the adrenal to the adjacent veins, special care and consideration must be given to the possibility of thromboembolism or tumor embolism. Compression of the cava can give rise to venous hypertension and obstruction with edema below the site of the impingement.

REFERENCES

1. Geelhoed G.W.: Adrenal tumors, in Pilch Y., das Gupta T. (eds.): *Surgical Oncology*. New York, McGraw-Hill Book Co., 1981, chap. 31.
2. Geelhoed G.W., Spiegel C.T.: The "incidental" adrenal cyst: Possible association with hypertension. *South. Med. J*. 74:626–630, 1981.
3. Aronsohn R.S., Friedman B.A., Turcotte J.G.: Blunt trauma to an adrenal cyst producing abdominal pain and anemia. *Am. Surg*. 44:605, 1978.
4. Geelhoed G.W., Druy E.M.: Management of the adrenal "incidentaloma." *Surgery* November, 1982.
5. Geelhoed G.W., Dunnick N.R., Doppman J.L.: Management of intravenous extensions of endocrine tumors and prognosis after surgical treatment. *Am. J. Surg*. 139:844, 1980.

14 / Multiple Endocrine Adenopathy

MANAGEMENT PROBLEMS

For the patient, the discovery that he has an endocrine abnormality that may have a very subtle connection to the symptoms he expresses or that may occur in the absence of any symptoms at all may be confusing. It is even more so to be informed that as an individual patient, he or she has multiple endocrine abnormalities that may occur simultaneously or sequentially throughout life. Furthermore, the implications of the hereditary nature of such disorders cause the patient to seek advice about how the rest of the family should be regarded and whether examination of relatives is necessary and with what frequency. The patient may even seek genetic counseling regarding the advisability of having children, questioning the probability that offspring would be involved in the multiple endocrine adenopathy diagnosed in an individual within the bloodlines.

The coexistence of multiple endocrine abnormalities poses a problem for the managing physician as well, since the simultaneous appearance of more than one endocrine disorder raises the question as to the sequence in which these disorders should be managed. A second question might be related to the appropriate testing to screen individuals at high risk for the other endocrine abnormalities that may occur sequentially during the course of their lives, and the intervals at which these examinations should be carried out. The physician will need to have information regarding the questions that will be brought to him by the patient about personal and family management decisions if a pattern of "clustering" of endocrine abnormalities is firmly diagnosed in at least one patient within the kindred.

INTRODUCTION

Endocrine abnormalities have been known to "cluster" within a given patient for some period of time. It has also been known that some specific endocrine adenopathies have a tendency to run in families. One of the original thinkers in endocrine surgery, previously mentioned in this book, was Harvey Cushing. In 1932 he noted that a group of cases he studied "showed peculiar and sundry polyglandular syndromes."[1] However, Cushing added, the term "polyglandular syndrome" should not be meant to imply that there was some relationship among glandular abnormalities that occurred for reasons other than reactive adaptation, since, he said, one of the glands had primary affectation in its activity, and all of the other changes were secondary functional alterations responding to the primary ductless-gland abnormality. This hypothesis may be correct for certain paired glandular malfunctions, as it later proved to be for Cushing's Disease, with adrenal hyperplasia responding to the pituitary overproduction of ACTH. At least one alternative hypothesis was also conceivable, however—that multiple endocrine abnormalities might be codetermined, particularly if resulting from a genetic or embryologic defect carried through several endocrine systems of similar origin. Support for this concept comes from the observation that the association of endocrine abnormalities does not appear to be random, but follows predictable clinical patterns in a relatively few recognized polyglandular syndromes.

The majority of endocrine surgical conditions arise from sporadic malfunction of at least one glandular system; these sporadic cases are of no genetic significance. When the combination of endocrine abnormalities occurs in predictable sequence within the same individual and then can be found within the family members, these hereditary clinical syndromes strongly suggest a common genetic and embryologic defect that might be understood, and the understanding of these patterns may be useful in management of the patient and family with these diagnoses.

DIAGNOSIS

Within the past 25 years, patterns have emerged that have led to a rational management method for patients and families, based on the proposed unifying theory of the APUD system discussed in chapter 1. At least three such basic familial patterns of associated endocrine abnormalities are now recognized, leaving open the possibility that others will be discovered as more potential syndromes appear to congeal into predictable patterns. One term for this patterning was "adenomatosis of the endocrine glands" (MEA) proposed by Wermer in 1954.[2] Another term used was "multiple endocrine neoplasia" (MEN); however, many of the members who otherwise fit into the patterns that these terms were meant to describe did not have adenomas or neoplasms, but frequently had hyperplasia and other forms of endocrinologic malfunction. For the purposes of this book, the term MEA is used, but is meant to stand for "multiple endocrine adenopathy," covering neoplasms, both benign and malignant; hyperplasia; and generally any endocrine malfunction that may occur within the glandular systems under study.

MEA-I.—The syndrome that Wermer described linked the parathyroid, pancreatic islets, and pituitary gland in kindreds that were later proved to pass the trait as an inherited autosomal dominant. The parathyroids were nearly invariably involved in the affected members, with early, mild onset of hyperparathyroidism, usually without symptoms in the younger patients. Family history frequently revealed in retrospect that older members of the family had died of complications of peptic ulcer disease. In the more contemporary family tree, patients may be found to have pancreatic tumors of mixed islet cell types. Pituitary adenomas were uncommon when judged by symptoms, but they were present at autopsy in most cases studied by this means. The later report of the gastrinoma syndrome (see chap. 7 for description of the Zollinger-Ellison syndrome) was found to be important to the MEA-I syndrome, since this ulcerogenic pancreatic islet cell tumor could be a part of the functioning islet cell disease in these patients. The diagnoses of hyperparathyroidism, gastrin-secreting pancreatic tumor, and pituitary adenoma are made just as they would be for the sporadic cases that appear in individuals not part of the MEA-I kindreds. However, an additional finding is that the polypeptide marker HPP (human pancreatic polypeptide) appears to be a marker for those islet cell abnormalities that tend to occur in the MEA-I kindreds.[3]

MEA-II.—The linkage beyond coincidence of thyroid, adrenal medullary, and parathyroid abnormalities came with Sipple's report in 1961[4] of an association of thyroid cancer and pheochromocytoma and, in a single autopsy case he observed, a parathyroid adenoma. These observations that Sipple made by literature review and overseeing a single case were later clarified when the thyroid neoplasm was found to be the medullary thyroid cancer which Hazard[5] described in 1959. Although these patients had parathyroid disease, the critical feature that brought them to physicians' attention was the pheochromocytoma, which in many cases appeared to be bilateral as well as hereditary. The later discovery of the thyroid hormone calcitonin originating in the parafollicular C cells of APUD origin allowed the development of a radioassay for calcitonin, which was a great advance as a technique for case finding.

MEA-III.—There is a distinctive subgroup of MEA-II in which the medullary carcinoma of the thyroid is very aggressive, and the onset is very early in life, usually spreading lethally before the patient is able to pass this trait along through reproduction. Although the pheochromocytomas resemble those of the MEA-II kindreds, parathyroid abnormalities are absent.[6] The other distinctive features of this MEA-III is that the patients have a very characteristic phenotypic appearance. The face shows prominent orbital ridges; heavy, creased scalp folds; large lips; prominent man-

TABLE 14–1.—COMPARISON OF THE FEATURES OF MEA-II AND MEA-III

FEATURES	MEA-II	MEA-III
Thyroid	Bilateral medullary carcinoma of the thyroid	Bilateral medullary carcinoma of the thyroid
Adrenal medulla	(Bilateral) Pheochromocytoma	(Bilateral) Pheochromocytoma
Parathyroid	Hyperplasia	Normal
Phenotype	None specific	Marfanoid habitus Characteristic facies
Inheritance	Autosomal dominant	Infrequently familial
Mucosal neuromas	Absent	Present
Medullary carcinoma of the thyroid	Variable, usually indolent	Aggressive, rare survivors to age 30

dibles; and multiple mucosal neuromas. The patients have a marfanoid habitus and pectus excavatum. The characteristic appearance of the MEA-III patient makes cursory observation an adequate indication for screening, since the appearance is so striking and so similar among individuals who bear this disease. Table 14–1 summarizes the common and different features in the comparison of MEA-II and MEA-III.

DISTINCTIVE DIFFERENCES OF ENDOCRINOPATHIES AMONG MEA KINDREDS

Although there are strong similarities among all of the endocrine abnormalities seen in the MEA kindreds and those described in the previous chapters dealing with sporadic cases, there are important differences as well. For example, multiple involvement is the rule *within* glandular systems rather than the exception. Pheochromocytoma is generally bilateral in MEA-II; *all* parathyroid glands are usually involved in MEA-I; multiple islet cell types may become abnormal in MEA-I either synchronously or sequentially in evolution over time. Another important distinction is that hyperplasia is a frequent feature of the MEA syndromes, rather than adenoma or carcinoma, which is the general rule in the sporadic form of the similar disorders. This has important implications with respect to diagnostic techniques, since angiographic failure is frequent without "tumor blush" in pancreatic islet cell detection due to the higher frequency of hyperplasia and microadenomatosis; a sporadic insulinoma is more likely to be localizable on radiographic examination. Because of the multiplicity of glandular involvement and the high frequency of hyperplasia or diffuse hyperactivity, operation in the MEA syndromes often requires total glandular ablation, whereas in sporadic endocrine abnormality, operation is often directed at simply removing the endocrine adenoma.

There is a wide variety of clinical expressivity within the MEA kindreds, and symptoms may range from asymptomatic to latent findings to crises, whereas the sporadic form of the same disease is generally more clinically consistent in severity. Suppressibility of the endocrinopathy without autonomy is not uncommon in MEA. Sporadic adenopathy of the same type is rarely suppressible. An example of this interdependency of the glandular systems is seen with MEA-I gastrinoma, which frequently can regress after operation directed to reduce the hyperparathyroidism that seems to be an endogenous stimulus to the pancreatic islet hyperactivity.

The genetics of MEAs appeared usually to be autosomal dominant traits in inheritance. This means that one half of the offspring are affected and that the sexes are equally affected without skipped generations. Although the penetrance is high, the expressivity is variable, and not all those who bear the trait suffer symptomatic clinical syndromes. However, the potential for physiologic and oncologic threat to life exists in all who are affected by this genetically predetermined pattern of endocrinologic disorders.

PREOPERATIVE PREPARATION

Although parathyroid abnormalities are common to both MEA-I and II (and, as noted, absent from MEA-III), approach to the parathyroid problem in patients of each MEA type is quite different. Cervical exploration is the *first* operation undertaken in MEA-I. Preoperative preparation for parathyroid exploration includes a screen of the patient's adrenocortical function to be sure preoperatively that a pituitary tumor has not ablated the ACTH secretion from the hypophysis so that a patient can generate the stress response during operation for parathyroid disease without acute addisonian crisis. The reason for this primary attack at the parathyroid level is that the pancreatic islet cell abnormality may respond to a reduction in circulating serum calcium by regression, as has been pointed out above for the case of gastrinoma.

In MEA-II, the parathyroid glands are the *last* concern. The reason for this inverted sequence is that the life-threatening disorders in the patient with MEA-II are from the physiologic crisis potential that is risked with an undisclosed or untreated pheochromocytoma. The diagnosis, control, and removal of the pheochromocytoma is the primary obligation in the management of the MEA-II. Second in order of priority is the oncologic potential of medullary thyroid carcinoma, which is a spreading lethal disease. Cervical operation is the second procedure performed, but the primary intent of such an operation is to perform *total* thyroidectomy for control of the thyroid parafollicular neoplasms. During the course of thyroidectomy, parathyroid exploration is carried out, but does not have the urgency attendant upon ablation of the thyroid gland and any regional nodes to which the medullary thyroid carcinoma has metastasized.

Preoperative preparation follows the same means of α- and β-adrenergic blockade suggested in chapter 10 for the sporadic pheochromocytoma. Analysis of the circulating polypeptide markers precedes the cervical exploration in order to use this information in follow-up postoperatively if the tumor marker disappears and reappears.

ANESTHESIA MANAGEMENT

Anesthesia management is not significantly different for the endocrine abnormality to be resolved at operation from that used for the sporadic case, with the exception that all patients with one feature of the components with an MEA should be screened for at least the lethal concomitant features. This point applies most specifically to a screen for pheochromocytoma in patients with medullary thyroid carcinoma, or for adrenocortical function in patients with pancreatic islet cell tumor.

OPERATIVE MANAGEMENT

Operation for the patients with MEA syndromes must take into account the multiple glandular disease and the high frequency of hyperplasia or microadenomatosis within these glandular systems. Therefore, in parathyroid exploration for the MEA syndromes, it is mandatory that *all* parathyroid glands are identified, examined histologically, and treated appropriately. Near-total parathyroidectomy is often appropriate for the MEA syndromes if indicated at operation, and patients operated on for hyperparathyroidism in MEA have a very much higher incidence of hypoparathyroidism postoperatively than the patients in whom a sporadically occurring adenoma is removed.

This precaution is especially important in the management of medullary thyroid carcinoma. Virtually *all* medullary thyroid carcinoma cases observed by the author have had bilateral disease, with multiple foci of primary neoplasm. Frequently the primary foci of the disease have been small, and the rate of metastatic involvement of the lymph nodes has been high, with the majority of the tumor burden located in metastatic sites. Since the parafollicular C cells are found in the lateral and superior portions of each thyroid lobe in the course of their migration from the ultimobranchial bodies in embryology, wherever these parafollicular cells are is a site of potential medullary thyroid carcinoma. It is for this reason that a "subtotal thyroidectomy" by the standard technique of an anterior dissection, leaving a posterior rim of thyroid along the recurrent laryngeal nerves and near the parathyroids, is distinctly inappropriate for the treatment of this disease. *Total* thyroidectomy is *mandatory* in the management of medullary thyroid carcinoma in the MEA-II kindreds. Advice for total thyroidectomy and lymphadenectomy in the paratracheal regions is even stronger for members of the MEA-III syndrome.

Similarly, exploration of the abdomen for pheochromocytoma should always take place from the anterior approach, searching both sides and all sites of the para-aortic chromaffin chain. It is inappropriate to operate based on the indication of a noninvasive test showing a mass in one adrenal gland in a patient who is a member of an MEA-II kindred, since direct observation and intraoperative stimulation of the opposite adrenal gland and all sites of the chromaffin chain are obligatory in operating for control of this disease, because the incidence of bilateral involvement of the adrenal glands with pheochromocytoma is 70% in MEA-II and III. If a pheochromocytoma is encountered in one adrenal gland and removed from the patients with MEA-II and MEA-III, careful dissection, direct inspection, and palpation of the opposite adrenal gland, with intraoperative provocation by glucagon stimulation, would all be required in the burden of proof to leave an apparently uninvolved opposite adrenal gland.

POSTOPERATIVE CARE AND DRUG MANAGEMENT

After a successful operation in removing pheochromocytoma, medullary thyroid carcinoma, or parathyroid adenoma in MEA-II, the patient is not discharged from follow-up if all measured features that were abnormal preoperatively appear to have normalized after the operation. All patients in the MEA kindreds and their first-degree relatives require lifetime follow-up. Catecholamine determinations can be carried out on an annual basis in those patients who retain one adrenal gland, in addition to the routine clinical checkup on blood pressure and glucose tolerance. Particularly in the apparently asymptomatic postoperative MEA patient and his or her first-order relatives, provocative tests in endocrinology are extremely useful.

Provocation is especially helpful in the insidious disease that may spread and cause the death of the patient before detection by any other means. For example, for medullary thyroid carcinoma, following total thyroidectomy, the patient may have annual determinations of calcitonin if no abnormality has been detected. The best way to be assured of extirpation of all C cells and their potential malignancy is by stimulation tests and calcitonin determinations following calcium, pentagastrin, and possibly alcohol stimulation. It has been recommended that family members of patients with MEA-II or MEA-III undergo postoperative provocative testing at six-month intervals, and high-risk relatives be followed up with annual stimulation studies for life.[7]

For those patients who have a recurrence of medullary thyroid carcinoma, radioiodine tracer studies for diagnostic scans and radioiodine therapy are ineffective, since these parafollicular neoplasms do not concentrate iodine. However, their presence may be evident by their secretion function even in metastatic locations. One method for selection of those patients who might benefit from reoperation is the simultaneous catheterization of the jugular veins and vena cava at the entrance of the hepatic veins and provocative administration of pentagastrin. If the calcitonin levels assayed are focal—for example, gradients in calcitonin attributable to metastatic disease on one side of the neck—such patients would benefit from reoperation, and a radical neck dissection would be indicated on the appropriate side. For patients who show simultaneous elevations of the calcitonin in the hepatic-venous effluent, such a determination augurs poorly for reoperation and resection of bulk disease with liver metastases apparent, and such patients might be selected for streptozocin and other forms of chemotherapy.

Patients with the MEA-I syndrome may be followed up postoperatively by the use of the polypeptide pancreatic markers, and there is a liberal indication for "second-look" reoperation for tumor reduction, although with a conservative approach to total ablation of the pancreas. Some of the products of the endocrine pancreas remain in balance even when one element of the pancreatic islet tissue has escaped in malignant degeneration. Ablation of the pancreas may not reduce the tumor burden, particularly for the disease that has spread far beyond the pancreatic limits, but it may leave the secretion from the functioning metastases unopposed by counterbalancing hormones from the normal pancreas that is residual.

FOLLOW-UP AND SPECIAL CONSIDERATIONS

Both the individual patient who is the propositus of the MEA diagnosis and the first-order relatives, particularly the young, are marked for lifelong screening tests to discover physiologic and oncologic abnormalities at the earliest possible and most treatable stages. This is possible for many of the endocrine abnormalities in the MEA kindreds for preclinical disease because of the distinctive tumor markers furnished by the endocrine products of these APUD-cell abnormalities.

The MEA syndromes have taught us that multiple glandular abnormalities may coexist within the same gland or glandular system, the same patient, and the same family. The clinical conclusion for MEA management is clear. When exploring for endocrine adenopathy: (1) search both sides or all glands for abnormality; (2) check the related endocrine systems in the same patient; and (3) screen the family members for similar hereditary endocrine conditions.

REFERENCES

1. Cushing H.: The basophil adenomas of the pituitary body and their clinical manifestations (pituitary basophilism). *Bull. Johns Hopkins Hosp*. 50:137, 1932.
2. Wermer P.: Genetic aspects of adenomatosis of endocrine glands. *Am. J. Med.* 16:363, 1954.
3. Friesen S.R., Himmel J.R., Tomita T.: Pancreatic polypeptide as screening marker for pancreatic polypeptide APUDomas in multiple endocrinopathies. *Am. J. Surg*. 139:61, 1980.
4. Sipple J.F.: Association of pheochromocytoma with carcinoma of thyroid gland. *Am. J. Med*. 31:163, 1961.
5. Hazard J.B., Hawk W.H., Crile G. Jr.: Medullary (solid) carcinoma of the thyroid—a clinico-pathologic entity. *J. Clin. Endocrinol. Metab*. 19:152, 1959.
6. Manger W.M., Gifford R.W.: *Pheochromocytoma*. New York, Springer-Verlag New York, 1977.
7. Wells S.A. Jr., et al.: The early diagnosis of medullary carcinoma of the thyroid gland in patients with multiple endocrine neoplasia type II. *Am. Surg*. 182:362, 1975.

15 / Summary

URGENT ENDOCRINE EXCESSES OR DEFICIENCIES

For the physician whose attention may be diverted from the important advances in endocrine surgery by the preemptory problem that concerns him at the patient's bedside, it is useful to be aware of the crises that require rapid recognition and correction. Many of the problems discussed in this book may be insidious in onset, of long duration, and corrected electively. Table 15–1 lists the crises that are most urgent in the author's view for the classic endocrine glands. With due respect for the ulcer disease and diarrhea of Zollinger-Ellison syndrome, the deficits that can be built up with WDHA, and the striking illness of glucagonoma, the author proposes that urgent crises dependent on polypeptide hormones of gut origin are limited to consideration of the β islet cell and insulin. Both hypofunction and hyperfunction of this hormone cause an immediate interference in the energy utilization systems on which the brain depends for its function. The endocrinologic hypofunction and hyperfunction cause failure in neurologic function. Coma on either end of the insulin scale must be recognized and immediately treated by all physicians who see patients.

Thyroid hypofunction is a serious but not critical deficit with rare exceptions, including the urgency of the diagnosis of hypothyroidism in early infancy. The life-threatening crisis of the thyroid gland is a property of its hyperfunction in thyroid storm. It is this abnormality and its prevention that formed a large part of the reasons for discussing thyrotoxicosis and preoperative preparation of the hyperthyroid patient.

Abnormalities of parathyroid hormone secretion can cause life-threatening crises on each end of the scale. Hyperparathyroidism may give rise to malignant hypercalcemia in "parathyroid poisoning," one of the rare indications for urgent operation in endocrine surgery. Failing control by saline infusion, diuretics, calcitonin, and mithramycin, emergency parathyroidectomy is still occasionally indicated. Hypoparathyroidism is also an emergency because of the tetanic interference in muscular function, with special reference to the muscles employed in breathing and in the myocardium.

Hypercortisolism is a serious disorder, but not immediately life-threatening, as is a deficiency in corticosteroid availability. Addisonian crisis may

TABLE 15–1.—PROBLEMS FOR EMERGENCY MANAGEMENT IN ENDOCRINE SURGERY

AREA OF INVOLVEMENT	HYPOFUNCTION	HYPERFUNCTION
Pancreas	Ketoacidosis	Hyperinsulinism
Thyroid	—	Thyroid storm
Parathyroid	Tetany	Hypercalcemia, coma
Adrenal cortex	Addisonian crisis	—
Chromaffin tissue	—	Hypertensive attack

be lethal under stress, of the type frequently seen during anesthesia or operation, and this deficiency must be thought of whenever primary abnormality in either adrenal cortex or pituitary is suspected.

There is no critical hypofunction in the chromaffin system, but the hyperfunction of excess catecholamine is clearly life-threatening. Pheochromocytoma need not be diagnosed or localized for the physician to recognize the signs of this hyperfunctional crisis, and urgent management should be reflexive.

Since there are a limited number of critical endocrine emergencies, each physician who sees patients might commit to memory the management methods employed for their control. Suggestions for management of these perioperative problems are listed in this book, and special attention will be drawn to the problem of hypoadrenocorticism and its prevention by means of a steroid replacement schedule.

STEROID REPLACEMENT AND STRESS ADAPTATION IN THE ADRENALECTOMIZED PATIENT

For patients who have lost adrenocortical function, a protocol is developed for immediate postoperative steroid replacement by the parenteral route, a tapering from the stress levels to oral maintenance of both mineralocorticoid and glucocorticoid, and instructions and preparation for any emergency stress adaptation on the part of the patient (Table 15–2). It should be emphasized that normal physiologic replacement levels of corticosteroid administration may be increased for stress tolerance, but there is no need for massive pharmacologic steroid doses for physiologic replacement. The patient's clinical status and symptomatic complaints are adequate for this exogenous autoregulation of corticosteroid dosages, and assay of plasma steroid or of the urinary metabolites is generally unnecessary. In the case of thyroid hormone replacement, guided by the patient's complaints, thyroxine, T_3, and free thyroxine index (FTI) plasma assays are helpful in titrating to adequate endocrine balance.

TABLE 15–2.—POSTADRENALECTOMY STEROID REPLACEMENT AND STRESS ADAPTATION

1. Intraoperatively or in crisis, the patient still needs no more than stress levels, approximately 100 mg hydrocortisone IV or 300 mg in circadian dosage intervals over 24 hr. Do *not* use massive pharmacologic steroid dosage for stress physiologic replacement!
2. Within 48 hours of adrenalectomy, taper dose to 50 mg hydrocortisone IV every 8 hr
3. While still giving parenteral steroids, give steroids orally at approximately 35 mg in AM, 15 mg in PM. As patient adjusts to oral intake, discontinue parenteral steroids
4. In outpatient follow-up, reduce to 20 mg AM, 10 mg PM, hydrocortisone; add 0.1 mg fludrocortisone to AM dose
5. Instruct patient in management of stress, heat tolerance, salt requirements, and use of medical notification bracelet or wallet card
6. Prepare "stress kit" for 48-hr parenteral supply of hydrocortisone if patient is unable to take in or retain oral feeding

ADVANCES IN ENDOCRINE SURGERY

A brief book focusing on the management of perioperative problems in the endocrine surgical patient will be incomplete and will reflect the state of the art at any given point in history. Pituitary abnormalities, gonadal disorders, masculinizing and feminizing syndromes, and gynecologic endocrinology are not discussed, perhaps because of the author's prejudice that limits his experience in these areas. For example, pituitary abnormalities do not often become life-threatening, urgent, problems because of their primary malfunction, but are reflected through adrenocortical insufficiency and to a lesser extent through hypothyroidism as problems with urgent impact on the patient with panhypopituitarism. Abnormalities stemming from the gonads may have oncologic implications for the life of the patient, but the physiologic economy of the individual is less disturbed than is the fertility implications for the species. In most endocrine surgical practice, the physician is called upon to be aware of subtle metabolic changes in an individual, link these abnormalities in function together in a pattern, and then infer from the pattern of the clinical syndrome the hormone mediator and the primary source of the problem. While correcting the disordered physiology, the endocrine surgeon seeks to correct the primary problem by reducing hyperfunction or removing mass lesions with the objective of returning normal homeostasis to the finely-tuned checks-and-balance system of endocrine autoregulation. The author has focused on the most common and the most instructive disorders of surgical endocrinology that are manageable.

But a more fundamental reason for the incomplete nature of a review of management methods in endocrine surgery is the rapid pace of advances in surgical endocrinology. New candidate hormones are proposed at an ever-increasing rate, newly described clinical syndromes without evident basis in apparent adenopathy or hormonal mediators, and an explosive crescendo in the information available on the biology of endocrinologic control systems will be changing the management practices in endocrine surgery rapidly in the near future. The translation of laboratory information to clinical practice has also speeded up remarkably as shown by the widespread availability of multi-phasic screening analysis, the increasing availability of radioimmunoassay, receptor studies being brought from laboratory to clinical application, and the evolution of the APUD concept as a unifying theory. Now the move of surgical endocrinology into the brave new world of genetics, and the study of endocrine derepression in subcellular systems, is suggesting new methods of management of endocrinologic problems. The steps from normal function to hyperplasia under stimulation to autonomous neoplasia may each be reversible if the control systems are understood. Many of the formerly fixed barriers between classes of biologic control systems that were either neurologic or endocrine have broken down with the discovery of amines and polypeptides in the nervous system and neurotransmitters that circulate as hormones. Beyond the endocrine glands that might be expected to secrete hormones, paraendocrine syndromes have developed from nonendocrine tumors. These tumors were generally of similar origin and visceral derivatives or near-neighbors to APUD cells. It was not long before the whole lexicon of endocrine mediators had been found from a single lung tumor.

Composite glands can now be recognized with different cell types, giving rise to different hormone species. The adrenal gland is such a combination of glands, but so is the thyroid secreting both thyroxine and calcitonin. The gut may also contain scattered cells of different origins with different peptides, some of which (as we have noted with somatostatin) may be paracrine in their effect in modulating secretions from their next-cell neighbors. The discovery and application of this information have given rise to a new autonomic system. In addition to the adrenergic and cholinergic, the peptidergic system has been elucidated, with multiple mediators. Several of the hormones and candidate hormones in the peptidergic system have been extracted not only from gut derivatives, but have also been traced to the CNS. These neuropeptides appear to be similar to, and in many instances the same as, the peptides in the endocrine gut.

Surgical endocrinology has straddled the basic schizophrenia that affected Harvey Cushing: both nerves and hormones appear to serve homeostatic functions, remain incompletely integrated in our understanding, yet continue to pop up in interesting cooperation in physiology. Many of these markers are easier to follow than to understand. But the considerable advantage of surgical endocrinology is that we can continue to follow the "hormone handle" on events that may be occurring without our understanding, and to use these tracers in diagnostic screening, detecting recurrence, monitoring effect of therapy, and possibly manipulating them to help control metabolic problems within patients. Neuroendocrinology has evolved within the past decade, without so much as a hyphen to stand between the complete integration of these two biologic control systems.

A reflection of the expected continuing growth of surgical endocrinology is the formulation within the past couple of years of two new societies for the consideration of these concepts: the International Association of Endocrine Surgeons and the American Association of Endocrine Surgeons.

CLINICAL CONCLUSION FROM THE STUDY OF ENDOCRINE SURGICAL PROBLEMS

The study of endocrine surgical problems is helpful in the understanding of the metabolic role played by amine and polypeptide hormones, and derivative from them, steroid hormones, and the excesses of these activities seen in clinical syndromes. The unifying concept of the APUD theory integrates the properties of the APUD cells, their distribution, their characteristic endocrine products, and the influence of these neural crest-derived adenopathies in clinical syndromes, both in patients with sporadic adenopathy and in those with linked endocrinopathies in MEA.

A clinical implication applicable in all endocrine surgical management is apparent:

If you find an endocrine adenoma, look for another within the APUD system;
If you find another, look through the family.

Index

P

R